I0876570

The Dance of Everyday Movement

The Dance of Everyday Movement

A Developmental Framework for Whole-Body Integration

Luc Vanier

Rebecca Nettl-Fiol

Elizabeth Johnson

UNIVERSITY OF ILLINOIS PRESS
Urbana, Chicago, and Springfield

Manufactured in the United States of America
1 2 3 4 5 C P 5 4 3 2 1
♾ This book is printed on acid-free paper.

Library of Congress Cataloging-in-Publication Data

Names: Vanier, Luc, author | Nettl-Fiol, Rebecca, author | Johnson, Elizabeth, author
Title: The dance of everyday movement : a developmental framework for whole-body integration / Luc Vanier, Rebecca Nettl-Fiol, Elizabeth Johnson.
Description: Urbana : University of Illinois Press, [2026] | Includes bibliographical references and index.
Identifiers: LCCN 2026024497 (print) | LCCN 2026024498 (ebook) | ISBN 9780252049972 hardcover | ISBN 9780252089657 paperback | ISBN 9780252049163 ebook
Subjects: LCSH: Movement education | Dance—Physiological aspects | Dance therapy | Mind and body | Alexander technique
Classification: LCC GV452 .V38 2026 (print) | LCC GV452 (ebook)
LC record available at https://lccn.loc.gov/2026024497
LC ebook record available at https://lccn.loc.gov/2026024498

The manufacturer's authorized representative in the EU for product safety is Mare Nostrum Group B.V., Mauritskade 21D, 1091 GC Amsterdam, The Netherlands. Email: gpsr@mare-nostrum.co.uk

In terms of bodily and mental skill, many human beings never progress beyond this infantile or quasi-anthropoidal stage. To pass beyond it in sport, craftsmanship, or science is a work of art. The processes involved in achieving the artistic sports, crafts or sciences are identical with those automatically followed in childhood or even before childhood in the womb! To cease achieving skill by well directed work during life is to die in that respect, just as surely as partial or complete death results from cessation of intra-uterine activities. Life is movement! Skilled movement connotes skilled living, i.e. art!

—Raymond Dart, "The Significance of Skill" in *Skill and Poise*

Contents

Part Four

Synthesis

Part Five

Applications

Companion Website

Readers of *The Dance of Everyday Movement: A Development Framework for Whole-Body Integration* are invited to visit the supplemental materials found at the University of Illinois Press website and accessed through the web page for the book. The site contains selected video clips relevant to each chapter.

The symbol ◎ in the text indicates a reference to these materials.

Credits

Video production and design
Kymberly McDaniel

Video camera operators
Laura Chiaramonte
Kymberly McDaniel

Video and photo animation
Hannah Hamalian

Photographs
Natalie Fiol

Photo and video models
Banafsheh Amiri
Oduwadamilare (Dare) Ayorinde
Veronica Bellon
Joe Bowie
Roxane D'Orléans Juste
Nobuko Graves
Claire Happel Ashe
Elizabeth Johnson
Ty'esha Lewis
Sojung Lim
Kato Lindholm
Nikki Marini
Rachel Rizzuto
Anna Rogovoy
Alex Tecza
Luc Vanier
Danny Yoerges

Children
Olykai Brownridge Fiol
Quintin Kucera
Miles Barnes Merwin
Clementine Yoerges

Foreword

Joe Bowie

Baking professionally is hard on one's body. Each day, bakers come to the bakery early in the morning hours to begin baking shifts that can last anywhere from eight to twelve hours. The tasks in the bakery are set, "routined," habituated, and narrowly defined: gather ingredients, scale ingredients, mix doughs, "stretch and fold" doughs, divide and shape doughs, and bake and cool bread and pastries. This sequence happens every day during every shift. Little attention is paid to the bakers (and even less attention to their bodies) who produce these delicious and artisan products. Bakers are not machines, but we are often treated as dispensable components of a larger production mechanism whose sole task is to produce products for our customers. Of course, this is not the image we see most often. We are fed a romanticized notion of artisan bakers honing their craft to make thoughtfully created, small-batch sourdough loaves and whole-grain pastries. I recall one ridiculously long shift. I had been offered a "big" baking job as a *sous* baker to help open a new restaurant for a prominent restaurant group in New York City. My primary duties were to train new bakers to mix, shape, and bake sourdough bagels. Early one morning, our most reliable and consistent baker fell ill, and I had to get to the restaurant in SoHo to take over for her. That day was also the "Friends and Family" soft opening for our new dinner service that required an entirely different set of breads to be baked. I worked seventeen hours straight without a break. My body screamed for relief, for momentary rest and recuperation, but I didn't listen. I had become so disconnected from my body that I had silenced its embodied knowledge acquired from nearly thirty years as a professional dancer to bake loaves of bread. "Hindsight is twenty-twenty," as they say.

I have left professional baking and returned to home baking, and I think about how different my professional baking career might have been if I had had access to useful strategies like the Alexander Technique and Framework for Integration. The phrase "to notice is to know" comes to mind as I delve more deeply and investigate their ramifications for both professional and home bakers. This phrase also speaks to what affects me most in the kitchen: awareness, connectedness, and body consciousness that create space for change and the art of "not doing," because baking, whether at home or in a professional bakery, requires "doing." If the information shared by Professors Rebecca Nettl-Fiol, Luc Vanier, and Elizabeth Johnson had been available to me as a professional baker, I would have remained more connected to my body, breath, ease, and overall well-being. I might have also more consciously dealt with (or at least mitigated) the effects of the physical wear and tear, "one-sidedness" that comes from shaping loaves of bread, and long hours spent standing in one place at the bench that professional bakers contend with during every baking shift.

Now, with this information in hand or "in body," I am a home baker who specifically uses the embodied knowledge that Framework for Integration offers to actively check in while I'm baking. As I make my way from the refrigerator to the mixer and then to the oven, I attend first to my breath, and then to my dynamic alignment, countering the static notions that accompany having "good posture" or maintaining a "strong core." I roll out a pie crust or piece of dough and use the Framework's idea of sending the *ball* backward and forward with each push and pull of the rolling pin. There is a newfound ease as I stand and sense the available lightness and buoyancy through the top of my head and employ the Alexander Technique's principle of *primary control* to free my head, neck, and shoulder girdle. I now fully integrate my head–pelvis connection, inherent rhythm, and my body's organic spiraling and double-spiraling. I toggle between engagement and resetting in hopes of undoing some of my habits and rediscovering the joy I find in something as simple as baking a batch of vegan chocolate chip cookies. It's not easy to keep track of everything, but it's certainly worth it and my body is profoundly grateful. Because, as I say, "Bakers gonna bake."

So, whether you're baking, opening a door, or getting in and out of a car, *The Dance of Everyday Movement* will become an invaluable resource for all of us as we continue to evolve in our lives and bodies.

For more about applying Framework for Integration to baking, see the following video of an interview with Joe Bowie:

Video: Interview with Luc and Joe

Joe Bowie (he/him) is an interdisciplinary dance artist with a Master of Fine Arts in Dance from the University of Illinois Urbana-Champaign. Before starting graduate school, Bowie danced professionally for over twenty years in New York City, touring domestically and internationally with two world-renowned dance companies: the Paul Taylor Dance Company and the Mark Morris Dance Group. Bowie comes to Framework for Integration by having studied the Alexander Technique with Professors Rebecca Nettl-Fiol and Luc Vanier.

Preface

> Even as you read this, some of our ideas have probably morphed, evolved, or even changed. We do not see this book as conclusive, unequivocal, or comprehensive, but as an exposition of our work at this point in time.
>
> —Nettl-Fiol and Vanier, Epilogue, *Dance and the Alexander Technique: Exploring the Missing Link*

This was written fifteen years ago as we finished our work on *Dance and the Alexander Technique: Exploring the Missing Link.* The last paragraph of the book invited the reader to "take the ideas presented here and explore them, challenge them, work out the movement explorations with a partner and see how they could apply to whatever you are interested in." Following our own directives, we have continuously and collaboratively researched, explored through teaching, and ultimately devised a more comprehensive system that both broadens and deepens the principles set forth in the first book. During this time, Elizabeth Johnson has come on board as an integral force in developing the work. Our aim was to reach a much wider range of people—movers of all kinds—offering a framework that gives tools for observing and analyzing movement, with the goal of uncovering and redirecting potentially harmful movement patterns, big or small, which may be interfering with optimal performance, whether in everyday activities or highly skilled movements required in athletics or dance. We call this system *Framework for Integration. Framework* because it is a conceptual structure that supports the set of assumptions, concepts, and practices that comprise the system we have developed. *Integration* because we are interested in moving toward a harmonious whole where all parts of the body and mind are related and interdependent, and movement is coordinated.

Today as we continue this work, the world is a substantively changed place. Discussions of what might be typically referred to as "health and wellness" have deepened and shifted as humanity copes with a once-in-a-century viral pandemic. Right now, what it means to be "well" is especially fluid. Themes of survival, rapid modern scientific response, and the politicization of disease, the body, and human activity's toll on the Earth's multiple ecologies are unavoidable. Multifaceted perspectives and the languages of inclusion and accessibility must be centered. To that end, as we have developed the vocabulary and experiential movement of Framework for Integration, so much of the research that was nascent while writing the first book is now fundamental and crucial to our understanding.

In research, as in life, there are certain unexpected circumstances that propel us into new realizations, changing insights and expanding what we thought we knew. For us, this happened just after the publication of *Dance and the Alexander Technique*, when Luc began working with veteran wheelchair athletes. The work he and a collaborator explored now defines the physioball work unique to our system. His two-year journey exploring how wheelchairs might be better adapted so that the athletes could have the fullest access and mobility in their hips and lower backs helped us to understand how so often those of us who consider ourselves fully "able" don't access or use what is available. We are excited to share more of this story and these discoveries later in the book—get your physioball ready!

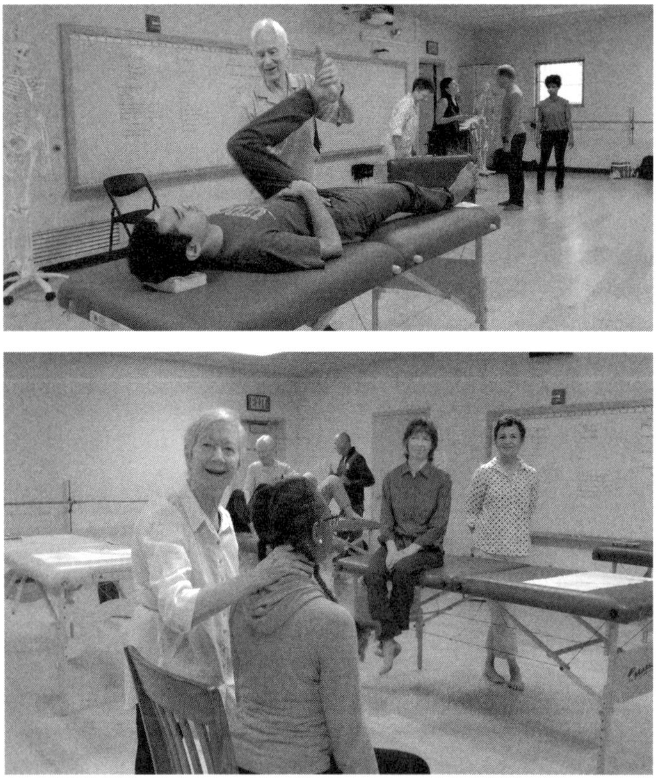

Joan and Alex Murray working with University of Illinois students in Rebecca Nettl-Fiol's Alexander for Dancers class.

Joan and Alex Murray

None of this work would exist if not for the teaching of Joan and Alex Murray, Rebecca and Luc's primary teachers, and by translation, of Elizabeth, who studied with second-generation Murray teachers. We continually attempt to unpack what we learned through Joan's embodied teaching and her approach to movement. Alex's interest in articulating F. M. Alexander's theories and the Murrays' collaborative work with Raymond Dart in the development of the Dart Procedures gave us a sound background for developing our own emergent system, which has roots in the Alexander Technique and Dart. As we developed and taught principles from our Framework in a myriad of places and contexts, those who knew of Joan and Alex's work often drew links and experienced similarities between what we were teaching and how it related to the Murrays' teaching.

A Brief Story of How We Got Here

In this book you'll experience a collaborative voice—the effort and process to integrate three authorial perspectives. Here we offer a glimpse into our backgrounds, each told in our distinct voices.

Rebecca's Story

I grew up in a family of artists and scholars. My father, Bruno Nettl, was a renowned professor of ethnomusicology, my grandfather a professor of musicology, my grandmother a pianist but also a modern dancer, and my mother, Wanda Nettl, a visual artist. My father's family fled the Nazis in 1939 and immigrated to the United States from Prague. Music of all kinds was prominent in my house, from Mozart to Carnatic music of India, American folk music to Native American Powwow music. My father's research took us across the globe, including two years in Germany, a year in Iran, and a summer on a Blackfoot Indian reservation. The arts, including dance, were honored in my family, and cultural differences were respected and valued. When I was seven years old, my parents took me to a dance concert by one of the most influential dance teachers and choreographers in Detroit, Harriet Berg.

And this is where my dance story begins. I was completely enamored and couldn't wait to start taking Creative Dance for Children with this wonderful teacher, whom I studied with for three years. We did modern dance exercises such as *chassés* with arms circling, floor work, and run-run-leaps across the floor. We devised complete works for performance, where Berg created the structure, while we created the movements. We also did research, cutting out articles about dance and pasting them in scrapbooks. I loved this class! At home, I made up dances for neighborhood friends, and we performed in the front yard. When my family moved from Detroit to Champaign, Illinois, having to give this class up was devastating for me. I tried taking a ballet class but did not appreciate what felt to me like confinement, so I quit dance class altogether. Later, I turned to gymnastics for the sheer exhilaration of moving in space—I loved tumbling and being upside down. When it came time for college, dance was what I felt most drawn to, even though I had no real training. Luckily I was accepted into the program at the University of Illinois, where once I stepped in, I was hooked.

My Alexander journey began in the late 1970s when I started taking private lessons with Joan Murray. I was attending graduate school in Dance at the Ohio State University, studying choreography and Rudolf Laban's movement notation system, Labanotation[1] (I eventually became certified to teach it and reconstruct dances from scores), along with Laban/Bartenieff Movement Analysis.[2] I was attracted to systems. I loved having a framework for understanding the language of movement. During this time, Laban's *Effort-Shape* and *Space Harmony* concepts were woven into my choreographic research and my teaching. I sought out teachers who embedded these principles into their work, feeling that my learning was enhanced by understanding movement principles that could be applied to any dance style. Had it not been for the connection I had been developing with Joan, and her extraordinary teaching skill, I would have pursued my certification in Laban/Bartenieff Movement Analysis. But since I found myself in Champaign-Urbana teaching at the University of Illinois, after taking years of private lessons with Joan, I entered the Murrays' training course in 1987, certifying in 1990. Straight away I established a course in the Dance Department called the Alexander Technique (AT) for Dancers. This course has been operating ever since, providing a lab for our local Alexander trainees to assist, and a chance for dance students to get hands-on experience with AT. And to continue my own development, I assisted on the Murrays' training course for many years. Lucky for me, I was able to drop in and participate in the course any time I wanted to until the Murrays moved to London in 2018, forty years after I had started working with Joan.

My university teaching began with a broad range of dance courses, but the core that began to develop was and still is my interest in cultivating dance artists with a wide range of expressivity and a rich movement vocabulary, performed with intelligence and elegance. To this end, in addition to dance technique or creative dance courses that are at the core of a dancer's training, I developed curricula that inform the student about function, such as dance anatomy and kinesiology, somatic courses including AT, and pedagogy courses that combine somatic viewpoints with technique teaching. Along the way, in the past forty-some years of teaching, I mentored students who were looking to expand their experience with anatomy and Alexander by offering independent studies, sometimes in conjunction with linking them to the Murrays' training course, so that they might earn their Alexander certification as they worked on their dance degrees.

Luc Vanier was one of these students. A ballet dancer who had suffered a back injury, he came to Urbana to train with the Murrays, thinking that he would need to give up his ballet dancing. I suggested that he join our graduate program so that he could train and receive his MFA in Dance simultaneously. Our collaboration started there, with independent studies that looked at the links he was seeing between AT principles and the developmental movement he was learning from the Murrays to ballet technique. Our work together continued, eventually resulting in our book, *Dance and the Alexander Technique: Exploring the Missing Link*, published in 2011. Elizabeth Johnson entered the dance program a year after Luc, and while she didn't train in the Alexander Technique at the time, she took courses with me and went on to certify as an AT teacher some years later. Collaboration with students is something I cherish—it encourages me to see things from new lenses, make new discoveries, go down new roads. Our team of three perseveres through distances, varying backgrounds, and at times, diverse opinions, to collectively come to conclusions that are always richer and closer to actuality than any one of us would have discovered on our own. For all my students, but especially these two, I am forever grateful.

Luc's Story

Physicality was always going to be part of my life. At four years old, I was already on ski hills, and at eight, I had my own little sailboat. Many summers spent in camps had me rock climbing, canoeing, and generally learning about how to live outdoors. I played soccer in high school and was part of a relay team that won a silver medal at the Quebec state race one winter. I always wanted to dance; in my hunger for movement, sports could be only part of the answer. In college, I even failed a project in a mime class by "over" dancing it; the instructor suggested Modern Dance, but at the time, I felt deeply connected to what I perceived to be ballet's clarity.

I started dancing ballet "late"—at seventeen—though as a male dancer, this is not atypical. I mainly studied with Daniel Seillier (1926–2012), who was the director of the *Ecole Superior de Danse du Québec*. In lineage, Seillier's main teacher was Gustave Ricaux of the Paris Opera, who encouraged him to study *port de bras* (ballet's arm pathways and movements) with Russian emigres Egorova, Preobrajenska, and Gorsky. Equally important—or perhaps more—was that beyond teaching the integration of how the arms function in ballet, Seillier modeled how to always treat the student as a whole person. He was never more interested in the acquisition of technique over the student as a unique artist. Another significant influence in my dance learning was Wayne Stewarte Newberry (1947–2014), who trained at the Royal Ballet and was also privately coached by Tamara Karsavina. Both Seillier and Stewarte taught me the importance of *épaulement* (shouldering), ballet's spiraling actions in the shoulders and torso. Stewarte helped me further understand how to integrate these specialized arm movements and emphasized the responsibility we have as dancers to pass on what we have learned from our teachers and their ancestors.

After dancing and choreographing for Alberta Ballet and Ohio Ballet, I went back to school to become an Alexander Technique teacher and earn a Master of Fine Arts in Dance—this is where my story meets Rebecca's. She encouraged and supported my research from the moment I was in her graduate classes. My passion was to link the work of ballet dancers with Joan and Alex Murray's developmental research (the Dart Procedures) that I was learning as I trained in the Alexander Technique. During that period, I also practiced various forms of meditation, which I still incorporate in my everyday dance and Alexander teaching.

I have taught people the Alexander Technique since 2001, and since 2011, have trained people to be AT teachers. One of the honors of my life was to coauthor *Dance and the Alexander Technique* with Rebecca, including a section on ballet teaching. Elizabeth, my partner in life and research, was a sort of silent partner in that undertaking. She and I often discussed the relationships between other developmental movement she was teaching from the Laban/Bartenieff framework. In the writing of this book, she is now an official co-creator of Framework for Integration.

Elizabeth's Story

Like Luc and Rebecca, I was a coordinated and athletic child, but I was tiny for my age. My mother shares stories of me being able to toddle fully upright under tables as well as able to Houdini-escape her grasp, running to climb to the top of the highest slide on the playground. In many old photos, I often appear to prefer being upside down (and I still do). My parents put me in creative movement classes as early as four and then drove the nails in the coffin when they took me to see the Ruth Page Nutcracker. I was a goner—it had to be ballet.

From six to fourteen, I studied in local studios learning what many white, American girls in the '70s and '80s did in such places: ballet, "jazz," and tap. I danced in local Nutcrackers nearly every year of my life through my freshman year in high school, when I finally got to dance the coveted main role of Clara (I swear I can hum the Tchaikovsky score from Overture to Finale). "Normal" high school would not be for me; I wanted to train professionally and be in a ballet company by the time I was eighteen. After acclimating to the world of ballet summer intensives and year-round arts school training, for my last years of high school and first year of college, I attended what is now called the University of North Carolina School of the Arts. There, I was taught by former professional ballet and modern dancers, most of whom had danced in prestigious American companies in New York. While my peers and I were heirs to rigorous physical training and important dance histories, we were also subjected to many cruel abuses—a legacy of embodied trauma still being untangled.

At eighteen, exhausted and injured physically and mentally, I "quit" the only fully physical and poetic way of being I had ever known. Through the gentle prodding of my parents, I found my way to university study, earning my Bachelor of Fine Arts at George Mason University. That journey saw me as an nontraditional undergraduate student, married too young, working, and with a five-month-old baby by the time I graduated at twenty-five. That six-year window of time allowed so much shift and healing in my understanding of the body and contemporary dance, primarily through study with Certified Laban Movement Analyst Karen Studd. Her intelligence, generosity, vast knowledge of the body, and deep embodiment of the Laban/Bartenieff work changed my life. I was stunned by how much I had been dancing without knowing anatomy or body mechanics or having a language to describe and critique movement. I learned how to improvise and choreograph and see dance as a field of scholarship and transformative creativity. Additionally, I got the equivalent of an English minor, which made me love and want to write as well as understand how literacy in anything can change a life. Ongoing education was how I could understand personal, cultural, and world histories.

My choices as a talented but traumatized young adult took their toll; that early marriage was rocky, and by twenty-nine, I was a mother of three. And here is where my story links up with Rebecca and Luc: At thirty-one, I was accepted to the University of Illinois to study for the MFA in Dance. The program put me in the path of educators and peers who would revolutionize my thinking and practice, shift my life's trajectory, and bestow professional credentials that had eluded me to that point. Professors Sara Hook and Dr. Cynthia Oliver treated me as an emerging artist, performer, choreographer, and scholar. I danced their choreographies and performed in New York and beyond with Sara's company, Sara Hook Dances, David Parker and the Bang Group, and after graduating, for Molly Rabinowitz's Liquid Grip. Learning to be a more skilled pedagogue under Rebecca's tutelage in her Dance Kinesiology and Somatics in Teaching courses set me on a clearer path toward my passion for somatic practice. Working with Luc as a peer and then colleague placed me as a witness to his transformation and led to our eventual life partnership. From my early twenties until now, I have been in therapy and interested in mindfulness practices. My formative years in the arts spur my interest in healing from trauma, the neuroscience of trauma, and trauma-informed education.

Beyond my MFA, my story includes having to create contexts to support my independent scholarship. In Milwaukee, where we raised our children, I established a small contemporary dance company called Your Mother Dances, where I made, curated, and self-produced my, Luc's, and other national artists' works. I taught undergraduate and graduate courses full time (non-tenured) while Luc earned tenure and climbed the proverbial academic ladder. As a woman with children and interrupted career opportunities, my trajectory in academia was delayed. I added certification in Laban/Bartenieff Movement Analysis (2005) and eventually became a certified teacher of the Alexander Technique in 2014 (Alexander Technique International) and 2015 (American Society for the Alexander Technique). I continue my "need to know" curiosity with Dr. Martha Eddy in New York, studying her Dynamic Embodiment system.

It is a curious fact that the only work which we really find laborious is that in which we are unskilled. Grief and loss accompanies the process of becoming skilled; once skill is achieved, profit and pleasure result.

—Raymond Dart, "The Significance of Skill" in *Skill and Poise*

I consider myself a voracious lifelong learner and strive to integrate the threads of my experience and education into all my teaching in dance and somatics. In 2016, after thirteen years of applying for tenure-track jobs, I was hired at the University of Florida, where I served as an associate professor until 2025. That opportunity supported me in ways I never imagined and propelled me into my next position as chair of the Department of Dance at the University of Maryland, Baltimore County. Grounded, I reach into the past to thank those who have shaped me; calmly, I mindfully observe the present in gratitude for all that has brought me here; optimistically, I look to shaping a future where human bodies and minds have better access to healing and integration.

We hope this book will help guide you on your movement journey as you discover the pleasure and confidence of newly found and heightened skill.

NOTES

1. A system for analyzing and recording movement. For further information, see Ann Hutchinson Guest's *Labanotation* in the Bibliography.
2. A system for analyzing and describing human movement.

Acknowledgments

This book is a long-in-the-making, collaborative integration of personal and professional histories and the oft mentioned (but certainly not clichéd) labor of love. To include all who, over decades of inquiry and teaching, have left their imprint on this work is not fully possible but here we honor as many as were most intimately involved in the project. As with the preceding book, *Dance and the Alexander Technique: Exploring the Missing Link,* first, we honor Joan and Alex Murray. Without their world-shifting collaboration with Dr. Raymond Dart and their insistence that the developmental perspective be integrated into their Alexander Technique teacher training, Framework for Integration wouldn't exist. Working on the book, we convened regularly in the city where they developed the Dart Procedures and on the university campus where all our histories converged, the University of Illinois Urbana-Champaign (UIUC). Thank you to the University of Illinois Department of Dance and the Krannert Center for the Performing Arts for access to the hallowed spaces where we learned, taught, performed, and made dances.

Many of the demonstrators for the movement exploration photographs and videos were UIUC Dance students and faculty; thank you for coming out in the cold March and warmer May to roll on the floor, sit on physioballs, be wrapped up in swaths of elastics, walk, ride bikes, practice yoga, pull weeds, and push wheelbarrows! Thanks to Professor John Toenjes for setting up our theatrical lighting and playing golf. Thank you to our intrepid digital media team: photographer Natalie Fiol, videographer and video editor Kym McDaniel, and videographer Laura Chiaramonte.

We offer immense gratitude to Alexander teacher and University of Wisconsin-Milwaukee colleague Matthew Ventura. Framework for Integration would not have emerged as clearly if not for his generous observations and graceful applications, which are embedded in all that is articulated throughout the various models. Thank you to AT training course director Karen DeWig for important dialogue over the years as we developed this work, and for integrating the Framework into training AT teachers.

Next, big thanks to our South American colleagues and partners. Since 2014, we have benefited from the immeasurable hospitality and generosity of Alexander Technique teacher training schools and private individuals who have been partners in deepening Framework for Integration, clarifying vocabulary, integrating the work into training methodologies, translating written documentation from English to Spanish as well as translating for us as we taught, and most of all, welcoming us as dear friends. We wish to thank: Violeta Winograd, Ignacio Gracián, and all teachers and students at Escuela de Técnica Alexander de Buenos Aires, Mariana Di Paula, Alejandro Schweizer, and all teachers and students at Escuela Uruguaya de Técnica Alexander, Merran Poplar, Roberto Reveilleau, and all at Escola da Técnica Alexander do Rio de Janeiro—Lúcia Bruce, Verónica Bellón, Diego Kantor, Sofía Cerdán and Diego Sefercheoglou, Marina Giancaspro, Nathali Rojas, Julie Cristal, and Kevin Litvin.

We offer deep appreciation to the Milwaukee wheelchair athlete veterans' community and Jacklyn Justus, MSN, the spinal specialist who oversaw the Zablocki Veterans' Administration Medical Center Spinal Cord Injury/Disorder Center when Luc was conducting research there, as well as the Buenos Aires–based mixed ability dance company Compañía de danza SIN FRONTERAS. With humility, we acknowledge that disability perspectives and studies continue leading the way to more humane and inclusive movement approaches and design for all.

We all received generous funding from our universities to travel, to conduct and present research, and for photo and video documentation. Our gratitude to the University of Illinois Campus Research Board, the University of Florida College of the Arts Scholarship Enhancement Fund and Research Incentive awards, the University of Florida School of Theatre and Dance, and the Vice President for Research, the College of Fine Arts and the School of Dance, at the University of Utah.

Finally, deep, abiding gratitude and love to our families (especially Steve Fiol, who provided delicious meals during our intensive work sessions!) and to our students, past and present, who are too many to name here. Over and over again, we dedicate this work to you.

Introduction

The Dance of Everyday Movement

> **The primitive joy of movement has been known by everyone at some time or another. The childish delight of hopping on one leg or twirling around until the world waltzed by us, may be for many a memory only of an order to 'stop fidgeting and find something quiet to do.' For others the joy of moving may have been disciplined by the objective satisfaction of games, the social intercourse of folk or ballroom dancing or the practical techniques of craftmanship. For all of us, movement is the great link between ourselves and every other form of life.**
>
> **—Jane Winearls, *Modern Dance: The Jooss-Leeder Method***

We can all probably remember the joy of movement experienced as a child. The delight of spinning around until we fell on the ground. The satisfaction of learning a new skill. The ecstasy of swinging on a swing at the playground. How can we tap into this as we explore and seek to improve our movement skills as reasoning adults? Finding something physical that is enjoyable is a good playground or laboratory for researching your movement. Relishing movement for its own sake could become a regular part of each day.

This practice of exploring your movement with a playful and curious attitude is a good first step. But without a system that provides a line of feedback against which to gauge your movement patterns, choices, and habits, you are relying exclusively on your feelings and past experiences, which may not be entirely reliable. Framework for Integration offers such a system, and we suggest it can become an essential tool for enhancing your movement practice. In learning this Framework, we encourage an interplay between lighthearted exploration and attention to detail—between willingness to go into the unknown and identifying principles that relate to your own movement preferences. We are not as interested in doing something well as we are in finding out how a movement task can be more comfortable, less injurious, more efficient, and more expressive, as opposed to more perfect.

The Dance of Everyday Movement

After *Dance and the Alexander Technique* was released, we received a lot of feedback from dancers for its relevance and efficacy, but surprisingly, we also heard from people who did not dance at all but found the principles applicable nevertheless. "It's too bad it's called *Dance and the Alexander Technique* because it is so much broader than just dance. I'm not a dancer, but it ended up being very applicable to me," remarked Max, an Alexander teacher in training. We were somewhat regretful that we were limiting our audience in a way by calling the book *Dance and the Alexander Technique*.

Do you identify as a dancer? What does that mean to you? So many people say things like, "I'm not coordinated," or "I have no sense of rhythm," or "I have two left feet." We posit a more inclusive definition of dance that could encompass the joy of moving:

> *dance*, the movement of the body in a rhythmic way, usually to music and within a given space, for the purpose of expressing an idea or emotion, releasing energy, *or simply taking delight in the movement itself.* (Brittanica)

Here, we want to open the door for everyone to realize their capacity to improve their use and functioning, to finding the "delight in the movement itself." In this way, everyone dances.

All three of us come from dance backgrounds; thus, dance is our knowledge base. What we have learned from dancing and teaching dance is at the root of what we understand. Even when applying the principles of the Framework to everyday movement activities, dance was always our litmus test. How does a baby rolling on the floor relate to a pirouette in dance, and how does this relate to turning to look behind you? How does lifting an arm in a dance gesture relate to conducting an orchestra or reaching to open a door? If a particular principle we explored worked in a dance context, we could feel confident about its translation to other types of movements.

Grace

"I want to dance just like you—you are so graceful!" said a participant in a dance fitness class that Rebecca teaches at a local gym. That launched a huge discussion about the meaning of "grace" and its implications to our work on the Framework.

What do people mean when they say graceful? Dictionary definitions include concepts such as effortlessness, elegance, or beauty of form, and moving in a smooth and controlled way. One can also associate grace with showing respect for others, to maintain grace under pressure and remain focused, attentive, and generous in challenging circumstances.

These statements about grace connote a kind of inner strength, the ability to inhibit an initial reaction to something, to show care for others as well as yourself, and to move with genuineness and simplicity. Each culture has its own ideas about what constitutes grace. Contrary to many common historically white Eurocentric views, we do not link grace to body size or shape, ability, or degree of flexibility. Also, we do not privilege one movement style over another. But we do ask, how can you move through life and through your daily activities with a sense of ease, flow, sequencing of movement, and focus? We offer a way into understanding grace—in the larger sense of the word—through a movement practice.

Movement Practice

Do you think of yourself as having a movement practice? We believe the possibility for a movement practice exists for everyone. It is easy to think that movement just happens and that we generally do not need to pay attention. Many of us exercise, work in professions that require or explore movement, or find joy in recuperative or leisure movement activities. If you picked up this book, you are probably curious about exploring something new in movement. It is beneficial to understand how we move as well as how to adapt our approach to movement at every stage of our lives and especially as we age.

When we say we have a movement practice, some issues that arise are simple to see. For example, it is easy to notice that when we do bring our conscious awareness to a particular movement, ironically, we often react by adding, removing, or interfering with the action in that simple act of paying attention. And yet, any movement practice worth its salt is most likely asking us to be mindful. We can also notice that while our bodies age, sometimes our feeling of our "self" remains set to the memory of a younger stage. As adults, sometimes we return to a sport, leisure activity, or dance form we learned as a child or adolescent with the remembrance of the body that learned it; if it has been years or decades, we may be simultaneously delighted and dismayed at our experience. We remember the coordination and ease we had and celebrate that we still know "how to do it" and yet, in an older, perhaps less flexible body that's lived a lot more life, it is now more difficult to feel fully comfortable or skillful.

So a useful movement practice needs to provide us with regular signposts and cues that help us match our body's ability with how it is feeling in the present moment. This realistically calibrated practice might be particularly helpful in rehabilitative contexts, say, after a stroke, heart attack, or injury. We believe the hallmark of a useful practice also includes the capacity to experience movement on a scale from the gross or large to the subtle, and from the simple to the complex. At times, this could feel a little regressive, like going back in time to an earlier stage of development.

A movement practice doesn't need to be "right," especially if we have expectations of success or perfection when we try something for the first time. There wouldn't be any learning at all if we always performed something correctly the first time. And though we know this intellectually, in practice, we are often very disappointed that we can't access immediate skill. Movement is a moment-to-moment lab, a daily practice where decisions can be made consciously, as needed. It is helpful to not be too precious: Sometimes we just have to go ahead and "go for it" instead of hoping to do it in the most efficient or nuanced way all the time, every time, or the first time.

Babies attempt many different versions of movement skills before those skills get baked into automation or habit. As adults, we easily get hung up on overthinking the intended action only to see our habitual reactions kick in over and over. In this case, the adage "just do it" might be helpful. Then we can notice what habits want to come up first before we try to change, even if we're working on a more unrefined level than ultimately hoped for. A movement practice can help you realize the impossibility of knowing what a movement will feel like or how it will happen in the future. What we can do is consciously set up the best conditions possible and then trust that we can mindfully negotiate the next moment.

About Development

"Why didn't you just tell me that in the first place?" exclaimed a student at the moment when she finally understood something that the teacher had been conveying to her many times and in numerous different ways. This phenomenon demonstrates the developmental nature of learning. Very often, you will not understand the entirety of a concept in one shot. There is need for development over time. Knowing this frees you up to explore without pressure.

We believe in the spiral nature of development—that development occurs in overlapping and interconnected waves that weave three-dimensionally, rather than progressing linearly. While we worked very hard to find a logical progression in the book and in the presentation of the Framework, please recognize that some aspects may resonate more easily with you than others. We do urge you to read the book in order, to follow the logic of how we have chosen to present the material. But then you may want to circle back in your own way, following your own interests and preferences to deepen your understanding. This is, in fact, the way we developed the material, by continually re-investigating, refreshing, questioning, and going back to see whether our earlier concepts continued to hold after we added more layers.

In developing Framework for Integration, we recognized this continuum of understanding and designed a multi-leveled, layered system that offers various lenses for looking at movement. It is adaptable to all levels of proficiency or comfort, both in movement activities that you might be exploring and your own grasp of the Framework's principles. If you are at ease with an activity, then the next level of complexity might be appropriate to guide or redirect habits. If you are new to an activity, the most basic model might be best for guiding the learning curve. The more you understand these models, the more flexibility you have in choosing which way to think about a movement or sequence of movements.

Keep in mind that in learning and experiencing new movement choices and patterns, you might feel completely disoriented, or just plain wrong. Don't be alarmed by this, but try to lean into the experience, realizing that doing something differently from the way you are used to will inevitably create some confusion in the nervous system at first. Also, you may find that our work challenges or contradicts your beliefs or previous teachings about movement. What we thought we were secure in may break apart in some way, and that can feel destabilizing. We ask you to playfully experience the movement explorations presented in the book, with a lightness of mind. The mind does not have to clamp down—you can feel comfortable staying in a place of not knowing. This idea of spiral development also challenges binary thinking and the ethics involved in the ideas of right and wrong. Rather than focusing on the "right thing," notice what you might gravitate toward, and use that information with curiosity, adaptability, and creativity.

A Guide to the Book

This book is a collaboration among three authors, each with distinct voices and writing styles, which we have attempted to synthesize. Ultimately, though tone and language may shift, we are united as creators and teachers of Framework for Integration. Our "authorial" voice often takes shape as a collective "we," but we also sometimes speak from a broader, universal "we"—our shared experience as human beings. In the movement explorations, we shift to speaking directly to the reader, the "you." We feel this approach most effectively reflects how we teach the Framework in varied contexts.

As mentioned in the Preface, we suggest reading the book in sequence, but we hope you will also circle back to previous sections to follow your curiosity or to clarify a principle. A Glossary of Terms is provided to elucidate our usage of specific terms and vocabularies. Most chapters include movement explorations designed for you to embody and experience the principles physically. We encourage you to try these out! Just reading will not provide the kind of learning that will lead to understanding this material. Some movement explorations are designed for partners, using touch or other forms of interaction to provide kinesthetic feedback, to gain information, or help direct a movement pathway. If you don't have a partner, or if you prefer to work alone, alternatives are provided. The photos and supplemental videos will also be helpful in clearly illustrating the movement explorations.

Part One discusses the philosophical underpinnings of Framework for Integration and outlines the developmental perspective in creating and teaching the work. Foundational philosophical principles are introduced, laying the groundwork and providing a larger context for the Framework. Parts Two and Three are the core sections of the book, devoted to explaining and describing the Framework step by step, with abundant movement explorations and illustrations. Part Four synthesizes the preceding chapters, offering a way to reflect on the ongoing process of change, and the habitual nature of movement. We include a chapter on applying the concepts of the Framework to the most basic movement of all: breathing.

Part Five offers reflections on design and practical applications of the Framework to a wide variety of activities, from everyday movements like raking, getting in and out of a car, and shoveling snow, to more specialized activities such as playing a musical instrument. Many of these applications were written by people who have studied with us at one time or another, making their own discoveries and connections to their particular movement practices. We hope this section compels you to try some of these out and to come up with applications of your own as well.

Part One

Overview of Principles

Introduction

Part One honors the root sources, foundational principles, and central themes that anchor and define the groundwork of Framework for Integration. The Framework synthesizes decades of our collective experience and transdisciplinary research that coalesce in a unique movement analysis system designed to promote discovery, adaptability, and change. Many of the following ideas as well as the Framework's vocabulary spring from Dance, somatic, educational, therapeutic, developmental, and neuroscience histories further contextualized throughout the next chapters.

All fixed set patterns are incapable of adaptability or pliability. The truth is outside of all fixed patterns.

—Bruce Lee

Chapter One tracks and shares principles from our major influences: F. M. Alexander, Joan and Alex Murray's work with Raymond Dart, Rudolf Laban, Irmgard Bartenieff, Nikolai Bernstein, and Ken Wilber. Developmental movement—the motor development of fetuses, infants, and babies as they learn to flex, extend, creep, crawl, sit, stand, and walk, as well as the evolution of our and other species—also substantially informs the Framework's design. We are indebted to many historic teachers whose incredible contributions have defined and continue to expand movement, arts, analysis, and therapy fields.

Chapter Two discusses the central themes of the Framework that have emerged over the years. We start with movement learning as the ultimate litmus test of human development and self-awareness, then shift to how we have layered the "lenses" of the Framework (Simple, Complex, and Integrated Models) to respect evolving complexity yet without hierarchy. Finally, we challenge ideas of "neutrality" or fixity of any kind when it comes to physicality and ideas of posture.

Chapter Three elucidates what we are calling the *infrastructure* of Framework for Integration. The Framework infrastructure is comprised of three "big ideas" or concepts that are consistent and interwoven throughout. Borne from the synthesis of theories and practices covered in Chapters One and Two, we call these building blocks: Engagement and Reset, habit and interference, and antagonistic action. All support the cyclic nature of work and rest as well as facilitate increasing body–mind awareness.

Chapter 1

Our Ancestors and Influences

To read this book and engage with the movement explorations herein, one does not need to learn with detail the somatic and philosophical practices that underlie the Framework's foundations. However, at the top of the book, we think it right to emphasize salient ideas that will recur, build, and continue to be resurfaced and revisited. While we highlight certain important principles, here we do not offer in-depth histories, nor do we feel it is within the purview of this work to meticulously critically and culturally contextualize the field of somatics and its progenitors. We are grateful for rigorous, more recent scholarship that grapples with the problematic lack of inclusion and acknowledgment, and in some cases outright cultural appropriation of non-white, non-European origins and contributions to somatic practices (Bradley 2019, Eddy 2002). Under scrutiny, few iconic historical figures emerge unscathed.

Between life's stimuli and our habitual responses exists choice.

—Ken Wilber, *Integral Life Practice: A 21st-Century Blueprint for Physical Health, Emotional Balance, Mental Clarity, and Spiritual Awakening*

We acknowledge the limitations of our lived experiences and personal histories. We cannot make ourselves other than what and who we are, subject to the times, national cultures, educational opportunities, and ideas of class, race, gender, and ability by which we were conditioned, and we actively work to bring to conscious awareness our inevitable biases. If any of the following practices, processes, or people in this chapter capture your curiosity, the bibliography offers many sources that have already laid down crucial ground, detailed systems and principles, and problematized some aspects of philosophies that haven't held up as well over time. As we document our influences, what most deeply informs our work is the quintessential elements of their theoretical investigations that have withstood the limitations of time and culture.

The Alexander Technique

Our largest influence and common sphere is the practice of the Alexander Technique (AT)—the ideas of F. M. Alexander and the ongoing work of his students. Early in the twentieth century, in his writings, F. M. Alexander proposed the idea of the *psychophysical* being. Throughout global history, many cultures never conceived of splintering the mind from the body. However, addressing the Cartesian body/mind split that came to dominate Western religion, philosophy, and culture, Alexander's proposition that things were either mostly mental or physical but never completely separate seemed revolutionary and new. The split is still so ingrained in our histories and current culture that while we might agree in principle with the idea of an undivided self, it is easy to engage in habits of mind that separate our bodily sensations and experiences from how we think about them.

For example, if we have pain in an area of our body, say our calf, we might refer to the pain as if we are here and the pain is "over there." We might say, "My calf hurts," segmenting the "faulty" part away from the awareness of our whole experience—my calf is not "me." From the mechanistic perspective of the industrial to the digital ages, we might also hope that an outside "mechanic," say, a physician, athletic trainer, or massage therapist, could fix that part directly without considering further the greater whole: "me." Like his contemporaries Mabel Todd, Rudolf Laban, Irmgard Bartenieff, Moshe Feldenkrais, and many more, Alexander insisted on the truth of psychophysical unity, often referring to the Whole Self. As we delve into the Framework for Integration movement explorations, attention to the unity of the body–mind is key.

None of the AT principles are inherently hierarchical—in teaching AT we move fluidly among them. However, the understanding of bodily organization does have a clear order and priority. In the principle of Primary Control, AT looks at the axial skeleton, primarily the head and spine, as the chief organizer of whole-body coordination. AT teachers "reboot" their students' general coordination and bring awareness to the whole, in-development person, which invites opportunities for freer movement. When we witness an adaptive, "just right" tone inherent in a coordinated body, it is nearly impossible to deny its existence. We might see it in action in our celebrated virtuosic athletes and performance artists or in healthy, trauma-free animals such as dogs and horses. This principle is at once noticeable and elusive. We believe the mechanism of Primary Control relates to identifiable poise—the grace to which we referred in the book's Introduction.

A truly distinctive hallmark of AT, not explicit in many other somatic or educational perspectives, is Alexander's outlook on human habits. Researching his own habits extensively, he surmised that long before we can address a task, we are already taking a habitual approach toward that very task; trying to change anything at the moment of action is doomed. Our unconscious, habitual responses to our internal and external environments often create difficult, cognitively dissonant moments in our lived experience, for ourselves and others. His solution to this problem was to challenge habits by employing basic movement tasks. In simple sitting down, standing up, and walking, he would move students in varying and unfamiliar ways so they could consciously identify when their thoughts and movement habits interfered with their desired coordination. AT teachers learn to do this consciously in themselves and help their students learn it; we call it inhibitory work or Inhibition.

Unlike the shame-based Freudian term, AT Inhibition is not an authoritarian kind of repression or self-denial but rather a refusal to consent to a habitually trained biological response. While this type of inhibition can be noticed in young children and animals (we love cats as examples—they rarely do anything on command!), it is not valued in Western produce-or-comply-at-any-cost societies. Pausing to respond to a question, sitting in meditation or contemplation, not immediately answering a text, or refusing to react to a demand or stimulus runs askew of a culture that wants us to respond with immediacy to outside and internalized pressures. Ads, social media, the news cycle, and traffic are chronic, constant harbingers of such pressures. There can be some confusion about Inhibition when it comes to movement—indeed, inhibition implies stopping something. Momentary pause gives us space and sometimes just a fraction of a second more time to bring a broader array of choices within our reach. Think of a time when, instead of being on autopilot, you took a moment to consider a small adjustment of your choices and experienced clarity and ease. As we move forward into the movement explorations, we hope this principle will help you observe how your movement habits serve or don't serve you well and give you a well-tested tool that will help.

In AT, Inhibition is partnered with something called Direction: a chance to redirect the energy of a habitual activity and then use it toward what better supports activity overall. This is often done through deliberate, conscious thinking while also refusing to capitulate to a habitual response. Traditionally, AT teachers might bring a student's attention to what their spine is doing, starting with the head/neck relationship and continuing down to the base of the spine (related to Primary Control outlined above). Freeing the neck at the very top of the spine where the skull meets the vertebrae is one of AT's prime directives. If the spine is freer, it can have a more connected relationship with the limbs and vice versa.

The next two AT principles relate to thinking, perception, and feeling. As humans, we are designed for moment-to-moment adaptation to changing environments, which now seem to shift faster than ever. What we understand as *thinking* happens in our frontal cortex: reasoning, executive function, social relationality, learning and recall, and voluntary muscle movement. Though habit is strong, we can develop the ability to bring frontal lobe function online to help guide the overall system. We need to think. When our body feels stable and safe, in a moment of challenging stimulus, it is easier to think. Alexander saw thinking as an experiential and embodied activity—not just a "brain" activity.

If we become out of calibration with our environment—or the environment itself is out of calibration—we are less able to feel stable or safe, which compromises our thinking. Our survival habits and internalized ideas confuse us, and our body's messages become garbled. Perhaps we start to think that a certain food, which is unhealthy or even harmful, is good for us. We misperceive our bodies as too fat, thin, weak, or unattractive when they are functioning fine, or we interpret certain words and actions as loving when they are abusive. These experiences are examples of how our perceptions and feelings can get really out of sync. Our map doesn't update appropriately; the script becomes skewed. This skewed perception of internal and external landscapes is what Alexander referred to as Unreliable Sensory Appreciation (original language: debauched kinesthesia). The positive spin on this human tendency is to appreciate how creative we become when dealing with our imperfect sense of the world! We believe our Framework provides opportunities to use this creativity in healthier ways, or at least in ways that hurt us less.

Finally, and because of our deep commitment to developmental perspectives, we mention AT terms called "Use" and "Functioning." Alexander presented his technique as an educational method with far-reaching ramifications that reverberated through the Whole Self to the greater community. He saw in his work a chance for students to effect change in all contexts through their general approach to or "use" of themselves. Here, Use is the compilation of processes at play in the act of living, which includes being able to perceive how you are using your Whole Self without overreacting to your self-awareness. Alexander put Use and Functioning in an interdependent, ever-relating loop. He insisted that the ways we use ourselves—consciously or not—affect deeply how well we generally function in the world. From the strength of our bones to our respiratory, circulatory, nervous, immune, and digestive systems, to our mental health, how well our systems function is inevitably related to how we use our Whole Selves throughout our lifespan. How we are or aren't functioning will affect our Use. Use affects Functioning. Functioning affects Use. From an AT perspective, no one thing changes without affecting the whole. Our capacity to think, inhibit, and make new decisions sets up a conscious process that allows us to continue changing, for the better, over time.

The Dart Procedures and Developmental Movement

For all three of us, our training in the Alexander Technique cannot be separated from other influences or past and concurrent learning. The way we learned AT was already informed by substantive references to and inclusion of what are called the Dart Procedures. And of course, we came to AT after decades of training, performing, making, and teaching dance; our contemporary and classical dance learning was heavily informed by other developmental and spectrum-based systems. All three of us agree that we gravitate toward and are excited by systems learning; we love the logic, overlap, and interaction of shared concepts that can be accessed through distinct but related vocabularies.

Reflecting our devotion to the Alexander Technique, the Framework for Integration system is process-based and not prescriptive. It's also developmental. We refuse to diagnose "problems" and, rather, hold that maladapted creative solutions need to be understood and redirected.

With the advent of accessible knowledge about neuroplasticity, it has become increasingly clear that our brains can change well beyond previously agreed-upon ages. Echoing AT's Use affects Functioning, what we think and do every day affects us more than we acknowledge. Recognizing our capacity for ongoing development throughout the lifespan changes everything. No longer can we think of our bodies as inevitably headed toward an expiration date and disconnected from our thoughts, activities, and communities. Aging becomes a very personal choice and responsibility and is directly linked to our ability to make new choices daily. Our capability to think influences how we age; we can learn to see this as an ongoing process, understood through movement, and available to us until we die.

Much of this perspective arises from working with the Dart Procedures, which are a series of developmental stages, outlined by paleoanthropologist Raymond Dart and put into practice by Joan and Alexander Murray, two Alexander Technique teachers. As we (Rebecca and Luc) trained to become Alexander teachers with them, something felt unique about their approach to teaching us how to observe ourselves. There were no expectations to grasp the knowledge right away, but rather the freedom to discover our individual paths out of habitual, unconscious movements. What the Murrays called "mucking about"—experimenting and failing as a learning methodology—was always honored and protected. This approach changed the way we looked at dance and allowed us to see its connection to developmental and everyday movement. Specialized movements were no longer isolated inventions but instead related to movement inherent to being a mammal and more. The Dart Procedures as we learned them are outlined in *Dance and the Alexander Technique: Exploring the Missing Link* alongside related stories about Dart and the Murrays.

Other developmental ideas that are infused into Framework for Integration come from:

- Movement sequences and exercises attributed to physical therapist, dancer, educator, and dance therapist Irmgard Bartenieff.[1]
- Laban Movement Analyst, Dance educator, and author Peggy Hackney's elucidation of Bartenieff's work, the Patterns of Total Body Connectivity.[2]

- Body-Mind Centering® (BMC) founder, occupational therapist, and movement educator Bonnie Bainbridge Cohen's Basic Neurocellular Patterns (BNP).[3]
- Somatic movement expert and educator, human health advocate, and author Dr. Martha Eddy's Dynamic Embodiment®, a unique applied synthesis of Bartenieff and BMC® concepts.

Laban/Bartenieff Movement Analysis

Rudolf Laban's comprehensive system of movement notation and analysis is a multi-layered model that helps movers describe the nuances and complexities of human movement and identify habitual movement signatures and patterns, and offers tools and choices for new experiences and change. Laban/Bartenieff Movement Analysis (LBMA) introduces polarity concepts in macro and micro spheres to map out an in-between spectrum without binaries of right and wrong or hierarchies of importance. Defining the extremes clarifies that there is a multifaceted range each person experiences throughout a lifetime. While there are named categories—Body, Effort, Shape, and Space—the crossover and connection of the learning is three-dimensionally expansive. Analogous points of reference exist across these categories—related ways to understand. For example, in the Space category, Laban defines varied ways people approach movement in their kinesphere—each person's range/bubble of space (Wahl, 146). One approach is called Central, where movement "radiates or penetrates between the center and the edge" (Wahl, 154)—think of a fencing sword thrusting from the hip toward a foe. This kind of movement also appears in the Shape category in Modes of Shape Change as Directional "spoke-like" movement (Wahl, 136). One category focuses on the body relating to space, and the other looks at how movement changes the body's shape; the lens shifts. Like LBMA, Framework for Integration defines larger, overarching categories or models, all of which are in dialogue and relationship. The Framework's Simple, Complex, and Integrated Models provide varied access points to embodied learning that may not click in one movement exploration but may be very clear in another.

Other vocabulary from the LBMA system that we have borrowed, and another of our main concepts, are the words *affinity* and *affined*. Laban asserted that certain movement qualities or actions were more likely to be facilitated in certain areas of the space around us. For example, because of the force of gravity, a powerful movement like a punch is easier to accomplish in a downward direction. Stronger movements can be anywhere in space—we can certainly punch a fist upward—but such actions are more efficiently accomplished when certain factors are aligned or affined. Along with that language would come the idea of something being disaffined—that punch up—which doesn't make something "wrong" but rather of differing emphasis. When actions are dis-affined, we immediately notice the impact or irony. As we have seen throughout centuries of protest and war, a fist in the air gets our attention—it also takes more effort and will to raise it.

Throughout the following chapters, we clearly define whole-body movement patterns that give homage to this aspect of Laban's work. We suggest that while no one movement is right or wrong, paying attention to the developmental and functional aspects of patterning and coordination may help us to make the most efficient choice for any given context. And for some specific and more rigorous movement training, knowing the terminology of affinity/dis-affinity can broaden clearer choices for high professional-level or expressive/creative movers.

Nicholai Bernstein: Development Is Not Directly Realized

The father of modern-day biomechanics, Nicholai Bernstein outlined his understanding of the brain's structure in support of what he called dexterity: the best creative solution to an imminent motor "problem." Concerned with how to best train athletes, his model of the brain's underlying structures included this developmental order:

- *Level A: The Level of Tone/Tonus.* Referred to by Bernstein as the "background of all backgrounds" (Bernstein, 116), this level "establishes the communication between the neural and muscular systems" (Profeta & Turvey, 4). Located in the spinal cord, "the first level's function is to prepare the movement apparatus to respond adequately to commands (influences, instructions, constraints) coming from upper levels of movement construction by changing the excitability of sensory and motor cells" (Profeta & Turvey, 4).
- *Level B: The Level of Muscular-Articular Links.* In the middle brain, this level "guarantees coherence in movements by controlling large choirs of muscles" (Profeta & Turvey, 5). At this level, "Synergies are shaped by the inflow of proprioceptive information about the whole body" (Profeta & Turvey, 5). The rhythmic aspect of movement happens here (Bernstein, 123).
- *Level C: The Level of Space.* This level "refers to how one performs a goal-directed movement in one's surroundings" (Profeta & Turvey, 5), and "In contrast to Levels 1 and 2, Level 3 can lead to purposive movements" (Profeta & Turvey, 5). Based on our previous experiences and the "interweaving of different sensory sources" (Profeta & Turvey, 5), this level generates an objective map of our surrounding reality that allows us to use our bodies in space. This level is the purview of Bernstein's *dexterity*, the

"capacity to respond quickly and adaptively to environmental demands" (Profeta & Turvey, 5).

- *Level D: The Level of Actions.* This level is located in the frontal cortex (Profeta & Turvey, 6). Generally understood as "sequences of movements" (Profeta & Turvey, 6), Bernstein's "actions" are organized in complex arrangements to achieve goals (with or without tools). The "different elements can be organized in different ways to achieve the same goal," because "there are innumerable ways to solve a particular movement problem, although each way has its own intrinsic organization" (Profeta & Turvey, 6). Typing and riding a bicycle are examples of tasks that, once learned, need little thought process but that also vary in individual approach day to day, depending on the needs of the movement "problem."

The neuroscientific field has moved beyond his model (even adding a *Level E: Actions for Expressions*—a task where movement symbolically communicates, such as acting or dancing), but we appreciate aspects of his foundational work. His solution to addressing motor problems lay in his sensitivity to and recognition of the mover's developmental level and the structures in the brain that could support the mover's goals. He believed that targeting direct change did not yield successful outcomes. Rather, if wanting a change, the layer above or below the target was best to address. For example, if a child is having difficulty dribbling a basketball, instead of insisting on fixing the inconsistent rhythm of the ball's bounce, we might pay attention to the child's sense of movement in space (relating to proprioception) instead. Rhythm cannot be present without foundational tone, and task for expression, which dance might represent, cannot be realized without first mastering general task. These insights are ever present in our work. In the three models of the Framework, one can loop backward and forward to address the desired change; directly trying to change something probably won't work as well.

Ken Wilber's Integral Theory

Another major influence that supports our work and clarifies our ideas of developmental thinking is Ken Wilber's Integral Theory. In his book, *A Theory of Everything: An Integral Vision for Business, Politics, Science, and Spirituality* (2000a), his general wish is to create connections across all fields of knowledge. Luc began working with Wilber's concepts in his dance teaching, most specifically with the *four quadrants,* with lines of development, and later the *twenty tenets* for developmental growth, which serve as a survey of the developmental philosophical theories currently available (2000b, 43–85). Wilber's work helps us understand with more complexity what is implied by the term *development* (2000a, 110–112). We translated some of these ideas into movement, pointed to similar relationships in the Alexander Technique and the Dart Procedures, and now have integrated them inside the Framework.

Wilber's greatest impact on the construction of our layered lens model comes from his AQAL, all quadrants, all lines: four quadrants that, when applied to our field, integrate all forms of dance into one schematic (2000a, 70). Applying AQAL connects dance, though seen as a specialized field, back to everyday movement that is deeply integrated into every moment of our lives. In the quadrants, the distinctions then become whether we are experiencing movement in what are called the subjective or objective continuums, and/or as individuals or a collective (2000a, 70–72).

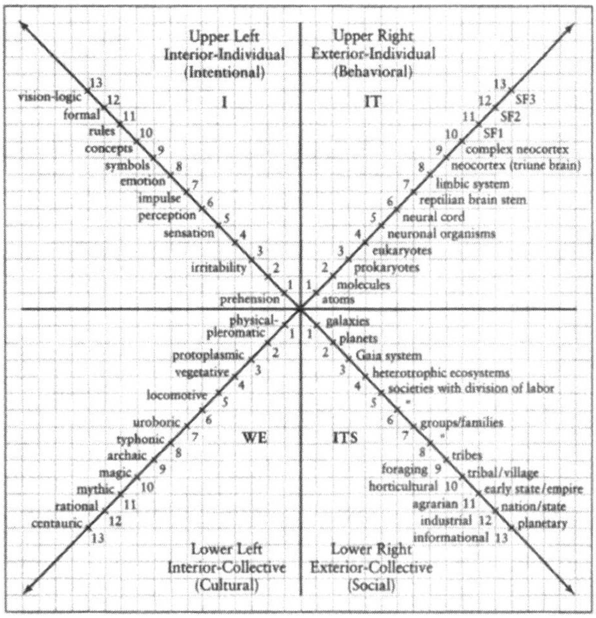

AQAL Chart (Wilber 2000a, 70)

An example of this vein of thinking about dance would allow a form like ballet to be related to contact improvisation—movement expressions that generally do not have a relationship or crossover. Both dance forms would also have connections to movements that fetuses, babies, and toddlers do and would ultimately be related to the evolution of the human species, containing references from single-celled organisms to fish, to reptiles, and to mammals. Inside and beside these broader objective relationships, there would also be attention to the subjective (what we might refer to as the *somatic*) experience of individuals, communities, and greater cultures. Our movement experience can then sit at the crossroads of these two continuums. We have both inner and outer experiences relating to movement, and we connect as individuals while also finding ourselves inside greater groups.

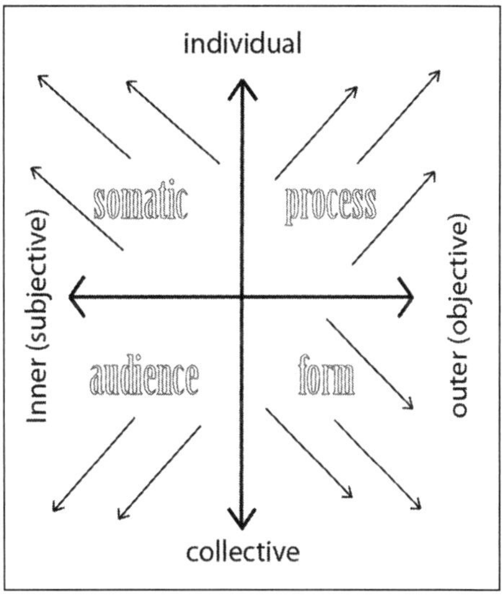

AQAL Chart relating to Dance

As seen in the above AQAL charts, two continuums—the objective/subjective and the individual/plural—create quadrants where one might find oneself enthralled with the process of training the moving body, say, working muscle groups in cross training (individual and objective), or deep in the inner experience of dancing at a club with a group of people (collective and subjective). Wilber also defines lines of development or evolutions that are linked to each quadrant (2000a, 70). For example, in one quadrant (upper left—Interior-Individual), sensation evolves to perception, perception to impulse, impulse to emotion, and so on. In another (upper right—Exterior-Individual), the brainstem leads to the limbic system, which leads to the neo-cortex. Objective, scientific facts (albeit ever in revision) are also juxtaposed against private, subjective experience to illustrate that existential *and* empirical processes are always in play toward a new state and a new stage of development. This implies that movement is not a static world of biomechanical facts and physiology, nor individualistic, ephemeral improvisation. Movement is everything: uniquely personal, evolutional, ever-changing, fully dynamic, and continually growing.

Wilber's *twenty tenets* (2000b, 43–85)[4] aligned with some of the work we were already doing with developmental forms (the Dart Procedures, Bartenieff Fundamentals) and pointed to the importance of centering humankind's capacity for development. We find frequent misunderstandings about what "developmental perspectives" means, as well as tendencies to overlay hierarchical models onto our developmental Framework. An example might be a value system that sees walking as more important than crawling and crawling as more important than lying prone on our bellies. And yet, without belly time and crawling, there is no walking, and as we age, we might benefit from going back to consciously exploring crawling. And though there are advantages to being on two legs, we must honor the fact that our bodies owe everything to our four-legged ancestors. Without them, there was no possibility to evolve to two legs. The tenets outline a world that is malleable, accountable, in relationship, and sustainable.

Summary

In this chapter, we have touched on our major influences. Our sources reflect recognizable crossovers and threads on varying spectra. Though unique and clear designs exist in the various systems that shape the Framework's ideas and practices, all of them:

- Hold to the developmental nature of humankind and our capacity to learn, change, and grow over the lifespan.
- Present principles and processes by which we can move toward awareness and conscious choice.
- Provide multi-layered structures through which one can access concepts that span a range of complexity.

In the next chapter, we will visit the synthesis of concepts and operational ideas that are unique to Framework for Integration as well as introduce our first movement explorations.

NOTES

1. The Basic Six: Femoral Flexion, Sagittal Pelvic Shift, Lateral Pelvic Shift, Diagonal Knee Reach, Body Half, and Arm Circle, as articulated in Columbia College Chicago's Graduate Laban Certificate in Movement Analysis (GL-CMA) program circa 2005 (revised language that references Bartenieff's work in her 1982 book with Dori Lewis, *Body Movement: Coping with the Environment*), as well as other developmental movement sequences under the larger umbrella of Bartenieff Fundamentals.
2. Breath, Core-Distal, Head-Tail, Upper-Lower, Body-Half, and Cross Lateral reiterated in Appendix A of Peggy Hackney's book *Making Connections: Total Body Connectivity Through Bartenieff Fundamentals*, p. 218.
3. See Prevertebrate, Vertebrate, Spinal, Symmetrical, and Asymmetrical Patterns throughout Bonnie Bainbridge Cohen's book *Basic Neurocellular Patterns: Exploring Developmental Movement.*
4. Wilber's Twenty Tenets appear in his book *Sex, Ecology, Spirituality: The Spirit of Evolution*, Book One, Chapter Two (The Pattern That Connects), pp. 43–85. Before exposition, Wilber gives his underlying definition of holons: "Reality is not composed of things or processes; it is not composed of atoms or quarks; it is not composed of wholes nor does it have any parts. Rather it is composed of whole/parts, or holons. This is true of atoms, cells, symbols, ideas. They can be understood neither as things or processes, neither as wholes nor parts, but only as simultaneous whole/parts so that standard 'atomistic' and 'wholistic' attempts are both off the mark. There is nothing that isn't a holon. . . . Before an atom is an atom, it is a holon. Before a cell is a cell, it is a holon. Before an idea is an idea, it is a holon. All of them are wholes that exist in other wholes, and thus they are all whole/parts, or holons, first and foremost (long before any 'particular characteristics' are singled out by us)."

   From Kevin Bowman's "Holarchical Development: Discovering and Applying Missing Drives from Ken Wilber's Twenty Tenets," as a simpler list, the Twenty Tenets are:

   1. Reality as a whole is composed of holons.
   2. Holons display four fundamental capacities or drives:
      a) self-preservation (autonomy)
      b) self-adaptation (communion)
      c) self-transcendence
      d) self-dissolution.
   3. Holons emerge.
   4. Holons emerge holarchically.
   5. Each emergent holon transcends and includes its predecessor.
   6. The lower sets the possibilities of the higher; the higher sets the probabilities of the lower.
   7. The number of levels a holon comprises determines its depth; and the number of holons on any given level determines its span.
   8. Each successive level of evolution produces greater depth and less span.
   9. Destroy any type of holon, and you will destroy all of the holons above it and none of the holons below it.

10. Holarchies coevolve.
11. The micro is in relational exchange with the macro at all levels of its depth (same level relational exchange).
12. Evolution has directionality:
    a) increasing complexity
    b) increasing differentiation/integration
    c) increasing organization/structuration
    d) increasing relative autonomy (increased capacity of the holon for "self-preservation in the midst of environmental fluctuations," i.e., agency)
    e) increasing telos ("the end point, of the system tends to 'pull' the holon's actualization, or development, in that direction").

Chapter 2

Central Themes

First, Honoring Movement

We come to movement naturally. From kicking in the womb to achieving our unique human bipedal stance, we reenact evolutionary and developmental stages that facilitate our growth as beings. Our brains developed in response to movement and to navigate its complexities, something that often seems to escape our contemporary understanding. Our species owes a great debt to movement. In our current Western society's understanding, movement is not held in high esteem. Virtuosic movers from athletes, to acrobats, to dancers are often seen as unusual human curiosities, sometimes worthy of special wondrous attention or able to galvanize cults of sports fandom. We tend to view them as exceptions and intuitives. In school budget cuts, after arts training, physical education is not far behind. In general, and despite much proven scientific research on the benefits of moving, in US and Western cultures, there is little agreement on movement's role in the general education and health of the overall person. Considering its import in our

The point here is that whatever patterns of movements we make train us to mobilize in the future whatever neuromuscular combinations we learned in order to make them. The movement patterns we make become us. The same is true for taxi drivers or scuba divers: whatever movements people make become the medium through which they sense and respond to whatever appears to them—where even that appearing is a function of the sensory education delivered by movements they have made. I am the movement that is making me.

—Kimerer L. LaMothe, "Recent Science Supporting 'Why We Dance'"

early, formative years, it's a bit surprising that movement is later left to "experts" or for amateurs to sustain in separate hobbies divorced from daily life.

As dance practitioners and embodied researchers, we center paradigms that often counter the greater culture and seek collaborators and studies that reify what we know to be important and true. As academics, we also have the privilege of finding research opportunities to work with like minds. For example, in early 2016, Luc was approached to collaborate with a chemist who established safety standards in his lab by teaching lab workers movements that would help them navigate surprising or dangerous situations. Finding research partners who are eager and interested in recognizing the importance of movement is generally unusual in our lives as dancers. Laban scholar Carol Lynne Moore stresses that once children develop language acquisition, though movement is ubiquitous, their awareness of it becomes quite sublimated (Moore and Yamamoto 1988, 2, 65, 85). Overall movement awareness and observation are rarely integrated into most people's daily experiences.

We wish to emphasize the importance of enhancing people's access to and awareness of healthy movement for every stage of life. As covered in Chapter One, Alexander believed *misuse* comes from the difficulty our minds have in letting go of habits and fixed ideas. In an AT lesson, simple movements in and out of a chair allow a student to notice overwork of the neck/spine, observe muscular tension, and encourage a general sense of posture in relationship to thinking. In much popular culture as well as in academic, and sadly, movement training cultures, there is often the premise that posture, not movement, can tell us what is going on (or in most cases, going *wrong*). Posture alone is a poor snapshot of a moment in time and is never the full story.

Many adages reference how thinking becomes rigid with age: "You can't teach an old dog new tricks," for instance. Neuroscientific research from the late twentieth and now twenty-first centuries recognizes a more plastic brain than was once thought, but those fixed ideas and embedded thought and movement habits often rob us of our capacity to change. An example is the way we might need to reread a sentence many times over when we used to be able to focus on reading a book without much distraction. Conversation partners might not be able to attend to relational or social cues and talk only of themselves, giving no space for the other. Rigidity in body thinking interferes with freedom and adaptation. Without awareness and choice, the body can do only what it does habitually once set in motion by a stimulus, and more so as we let it unconsciously repeat a pattern time and time again.

The ability to bring habitual movement patterns to conscious awareness and redirect them is what this book is all about, and more specifically, redirecting in a manner that brings joy, simplicity, and ultimately, greater freedom. One of the main challenges of working with the body is how easy it is to judge and categorize our movements in ways that bring less joy, more confusion, and stubborn commitment to ideas that continue not to work for us. Were toddlers to approach movement this way, they would never be able to stand up.

The Layered Lens Model

Inspired by Joan and Alex Murray and Raymond Dart's work, we built the Framework to correlate with a developmental path while simultaneously honoring that the path is in no way linear. At every learning stage, we move forward and then regress, grasp large general concepts, and then circle back to refine them. As we go one step backward to stand more confidently in our knowing, we gain the stability and courage needed to leap ahead to something more challenging.

The Framework is comprised of three distinct yet overlapping models: Simple, Complex, and Integrated. We advocate approaching the models as lenses that can provide varied but aligned perspectives—all guide the mover toward coordinated, integrated movement. There is no one path for everyone, and the Framework is meant to provide a structure for understanding and exploration. All the models are applicable to all movement at all levels of ability.

A clear example of the layered lens structure can be found in what is known as Laban's Dimensional Scale,[1] based on one of the fundamental structures of geometric thinking, the dimensional cross. Here, height (verticality), width (horizontality), and depth (sagittal-ness) intersect. The "scale" is a simple, embodied tracing of three-dimensionality. One can perform this with the whole body or parts of the body, seated or standing, and once the pattern is learned and repeatable, other concepts can be layered over the structure. The movement defines the three cardinal dimensions. The mover explores the space reaching above the head and down to the floor (vertical), side to side (horizontal), and the space behind and in front of the body (sagittal), leading with one arm and then the other.

- Layer I: The three dimensions can be moved as a spatial exercise only. Find the pattern in *space*. The "where."
- Layer II: Each area in space connotes a kind of movement quality layered onto the spatial idea, such as: Going up in the vertical dimension is layered with a quality of lightness. You are accurate in the space as well as the specific quality. The "how."
- Layer III: Each area in space connotes a way that the body shapes. This layer no longer emphasizes movement qualities but rather how the body changes shape. For example, going up in the vertical dimension, no longer think about the lightness of movement. Instead, think about and embody how the body rises. The "what."

See the link below for a fully illustrated version and observe how the movement experience changes in response to each lens. If so desired, you can try this out as a movement exploration!

Video: Laban's Dimensional Scale

If you did this as a movement exploration, you may have noticed that though each repetition of the scale goes through the same movements in space, when we layer our thinking, we may discover more physical sensations, emotions, and details about what we are doing. No one way of approaching the scale is "correct" or better than the other. Each lens shifts attention to a specific and yet complementary way of thinking. Inside each, we can notice our preferences and habits. Maybe you enjoyed rising more than sinking or the quality of speeding up over slowing down. Perhaps this exploration brought some awareness to preferences that may be at play throughout your daily activities. You likely have "go-to" movement strategies. While they might work most of the time, sometimes movement habits cause trouble or confusion. Having multiple ways to identify "what's going on" can provide inroads to seeing ourselves honestly as well as offer ways to see more possibilities. Inspired by LBMA, the Framework employs this layered approach through all the models.

Challenging "Neutral"

Biomechanical and anatomical models of human posture often posit a *place* of nonmoving equilibrium—a static, correct way to stand, sit, or lie down—called "neutral." We refute this static model that seeks to find the "right" shape or prescribe a "correct" relationship among body parts.

MOVEMENT EXPLORATION 2.1: NO NEUTRAL

Sit upright in a chair balanced on your sit bones, with both feet on the floor. Now look around to see what is behind you, allowing yourself to shift your weight as you look around. Then let go of that and let yourself come back to sitting facing forward. Do the same going the other way.

Once you have experienced this spiral in both directions and returned to your original orientation, you might notice, in a subtle or not-so-subtle way, that you feel a little bit different now. You may notice a feeling of more mobility and ease. In any case, you are now in a renewed position, rather than a "neutral" one. You are not coming back to a known place, but rather, you have discovered a newly reorganized place.

We deconstruct the idea that there is such a thing as "neutral" when it comes to upright bipedal human posture or body parts, for example, the spine, pelvis, or feet.

We are not searching for a neutral spine, neutral pelvis, or neutral posture. Our explorations are more dynamic, recognizing that we are always moving, always coming from somewhere to go somewhere, even when seemingly stationary. We stopped looking for the place of origin, the zero, or the symmetry of coming back to something prescribed. We replaced the idea of neutral with:

- Inner and outer relationships.
- An understanding of being on a developmental spectrum.
- Welcoming the unknown.
- Moving away from the comfort of old ideas toward three-dimensionality.
- Moving toward rhythmic integration—a step further than dynamic alignment.

The idea that there is a fixed place that is neutral—neither here nor there, with our "gears" disconnected from our "parts"—is too static and mechanical a model for living, moving beings. Dismissing neutrality as an organizing principle gives us the freedom to explore.

NOTES

1. For more information about the Laban Framework, see Appendix A, "A Brief Overview of the Framework of Laban Movement Analysis," in Peggy Hackney's *Making Connections: Total Body Integration Through Bartenieff Fundamentals.* The spatial reference for the dimensional cross on which the Dimensional Scale is based is on p. 224. More on the Dimensional Scale and the related Defense Scale can be found on pp. 270–274 of *Actor Training the Laban Way: An Integrated Approach to Voice, Speech, and Movement,* by Barbara Adrian.

Chapter 3

Infrastructure

> **Our language is singularly lacking in a terminology of muscle movement and its memory.**
>
> **—Raymond Dart, "The Significance of Skill," from *Skill and Poise***

Building a Vocabulary

Three important concepts provide the building blocks that support Framework for Integration. A key component is what we have chosen to call *Engagement and Reset.* The idea is that all movement can be seen as being composed of action (Engagement) and letting go of that action (Reset). The second concept is *Habit and Interference,* recognizing that each of us has a unique set of movement patterns and habits, and the Framework is designed to give us a system to help us recognize and, if desired, redirect these habits. And the third foundational concept is Alexander's *Antagonistic Action,* an aspect of tone that elicits coordination. These constructs provide a scaffold as we build and outline the models in the following chapters.

> **In every game and craft, perfect relaxation of the unwanted muscles is the key to skilled performance.**
>
> **—Raymond Dart, "The Significance of Skill," from *Skill and Poise***

Engagement and Reset

If a muscle engages, it must eventually let go. Coordinated movement relies on discovering the interplay between Engagement and Reset. We can notice whether we are Engaging our musculature in every movement, never allowing a Reset to occur, or whether we are too relaxed with not enough tone to efficiently launch the movement. These terms will be further elucidated throughout the chapters in Parts Three and Four, but a simple illustration for this is a baby lying prone and then looking around his right shoulder to see his mother (Engagement), to end up rolling onto his back (Reset). Intent is an important aspect of this. The baby has a desire to see his mother—it is not an abstract movement. Aligning activity and intent, and noticing the way they may become disassociated, allows us to find relationships in the movement that promote greater ease.

Reset should not be confused with relaxing. Relaxing can imply releasing or collapsing, but the sense of passivity implied in the word relax is not what we are looking for in our concept of Reset. Ideas such as adjusting, reevaluating, and allowing space and opportunity for making changes are present in the word Reset. At one time we considered using the word "refresh," the button you click on the computer that gives you the most recent version of the page you are viewing. When a webpage refreshes, it updates, collecting and integrating all the new information. But we settled on Reset to consider finding something new. Resetting is to be differentiated from the idea that the activity returns to a neutral place.

Allowing ourselves to fully explore one end of a spectrum will usually lead to finding what the other is about. For example, a full Reset will often lead to the restarting of Engagements, and vice versa. The interchange of Engagement and Reset gives movement a rhythmic phrasing and encourages resilience. This will be discussed with greater depth in Chapter Six, Timing Matters.

Habit and Interference

The second basic theme deals with habit and interference. It is not enough to learn a series of movements or exercises, but rather to determine the *way* you are doing these movements. Habituated movements feel "normal" to us. We need a way of finding out how we are doing what we are doing, and whether the "how" is appropriate. As we pay attention, we can begin to tease out the interferences of our habits in relation to what we are aiming to do. Since everyone is different and each of us has a unique way of moving, giving the same movement instruction to everyone does not address the individual variations involved in performing the movement.

Change involves carrying out an activity against the habit of life.

—F. M. Alexander, *The Alexander Technique: The Essential Writings of F. Matthias Alexander*

The Framework can serve as a movement pattern recognition system, from simple to complex, and can help us to figure out what our movement habits are and how they may interfere with functioning. Movement is not just movement. It involves our whole body and mind and all aspects of our being. We all have a personal movement signature, but the challenge is finding a way to objectively look at our movement patterns with an eye toward finding the best movement choices or responses at any given moment.

Inspired by Wilber's Integral Theory, we propose that habits are not something to be broken, to be left behind and replaced by newer shiny ones, but rather, to be deeply known first, and next understood as a fascinating creative response. For example, we can reframe the way we think about injuries. Sometimes our creativity goes rogue and our habits run unchecked. When we get hurt, we need more support to make better decisions. We do not want to make our habits our enemies; indeed, habits support our capacity to take action, they support our *will* to take action, and not much gets done without them. Certain habits align with certain physical and mental tendencies that, once recognized, can be redirected. In a perfect world, stopping habitual responses would allow us to find new, creative ones (inhibition). The rub is: Our sense of what feels right is often so strong that it overrides our ability to redirect.

The Framework offers a series of stepping stones toward more choices and, ultimately, a system against which to gauge your movement preferences. For example, if you begin to notice that your back hurts after you have been raking leaves, what is to be done? A typical approach might be to stretch the part bothering you or to think that you may need to build some strength in a part of the body. Both approaches might be beneficial, but first it would be useful to take a look and see what you are doing with yourself as you rake. Are you able to recognize how your usual habits are affecting the raking? For example, are you overly extending the rake, arching your back, and then leaving it arched as you bring the leaves toward you? Or is your habit to round your back and leave it that way for both phases of the raking? Once you have explored the Simple Model in the Framework, you will have a language for looking at your habits in relationship to this activity. We hope you will be able to make new, simpler decisions, beyond stretching and building muscle, or trying to hold a correct posture.

Habits of thinking and moving can affect the coordination of our functioning. We refer to these as *interferences*. We prefer this language to "good" and "bad" habits, and/or the thought of having to break habits. We would like to reframe this notion and recognize our habits as an opportunity for curiosity rather than judgment.

Antagonistic Action

The word "antagonistic" in descriptive language often bears a negative connotation suggesting hostility and conflict. But in relationship to movement contexts, and as in the quote on the next page, *antagonistic* refers rather to a dynamic interaction of opposing muscle groups in relationship to gravity. The support, grounding, stability, and balance that come from that relationship can now positively reframe this term. In Alexander Technique, we often work to elicit the antagonistic action that encourages a balance in the opposing muscles, a phenomenon that Alexander described as "positions of mechanical advantage" (Alexander 1996, 118). In the Framework, we extend this idea further in assessing a way to find support in one aspect of the whole body to allow another to free up and move (also related to the Laban/Bartenieff paradigm of Stability and Mobility) (Wahl 2019, 39–40). Another way to think about it is in terms of connectivity. Finding the connections between specific parts of the body can serve to support the movement of other parts. The Framework rests on the proposal that antagonistic action is clearly experienced in the double-spiral musculature of the body, where the spirals work both together and in opposition to create overlapping layers of movement, support, and tone (see Chapter Five, the Complex Model). Chapters Eight and Nine address antagonistic action more thoroughly through the application of imaginary upper and lower triangles in the body. Antagonistic action is balancing simultaneous Engagements and Resets throughout constellations of bodily relationships.

I remember that I was very interested in the lengthening in the front of the neck and torso. What I was always watching, of course, was the antagonistic action. Observing the antagonistic action helped me to understand how to bring about lengthening and widening. Early on, Alexander called antagonistic action "the great principle."

—Joan Murray, *Beginning from the Beginning*

Part Two

Framework for Integration, Simple and Complex Models

Introduction

In looking back on the system's development, we were determined to make the principles of the Alexander Technique relevant and available for teaching dancers. Learning the Dart Procedures from the Murrays provided an important missing link. Over twenty years, we have continued to research the Dart Procedures for the purpose of creating a language that can communicate what we saw at play when Joan and Alex were working. As we scrutinized the movement sequencing in the Dart Procedures, sometimes repeating or staying in one part for a good while, we began distilling these moments and patterns into a coherent shorthand. Our work with dancers, wheelchair athletes, private students from all walks of life, and Alexander Technique teachers and trainees was the testing ground and embodied laboratory for developing Framework for Integration, which we now apply to a broad spectrum of movement.

Framework for Integration comprises three interwoven models. Each model provides a lens with which to observe and analyze movement. The *Simple Model* looks at the two basic curves of the body: Primary, which is the curve we were born in, and its opposite, Secondary, which takes us out of self and into the world. In this model, we do not look simply at a shape or position, but rather at movement and intention, and the interplay of Primary and Secondary in action. The *Complex Model* recognizes our double-spiral musculature, reflecting the human body's three-dimensional design. Understanding this complex diagonal interweaving of Primary and Secondary curves throughout the body clearly illustrates how movement of any part affects the movement of the whole. The *Integrated Model* looks at the relationship and responsiveness of the hips to the head and the head to the hips, further delineating the interplay of engaging in and releasing from activity. We also describe two overlapping and three-dimensional triangles that function in opposition to each other, providing the antagonistic action that elicits resilience and support.

Within each model, we look more closely at the concepts of Engagement: actively investing yourself into a movement with intention and direction, and Resetting: letting go of that engagement, or undoing. In coordinated movement, we see fluctuation between these two activities. In uncoordinated movement, we may notice overexertion for every movement (too much Engagement with not enough Reset, for example, continuing to grasp with excess tension the lid of a jar of pickles after it's open), or an emphasis on relaxing or passivity (not enough Engagement and too much Reset, for example, arms hanging limply at your sides while walking). This interaction of Engagements and Resets becomes more complex as we apply them from one model to another.

All three models are equally important and exist simultaneously, but they can be described and viewed separately, ultimately allowing us to see whether our tendencies or movement patterns take us toward or away from integration and giving us strategies that lead us toward better use. In other words, we could take a movement example and look at it from any of these models—we don't necessarily look for which one to use, but rather, we realize that we can see things from multiple viewpoints. This multilayered framework is adaptable and expandable, and it recognizes the intricate design of the whole human organism. Our aim is to provide a system that offers tools for recognizing movement habits and potential interferences with good coordination, while providing clear strategies for redirecting toward better integration.

In Part Two, we focus on the Simple and Complex Models. As mentioned in the Introduction to the book, you are encouraged to get up and move! The Movement Explorations and accompanying photos and videos are designed to teach the principles in these models experientially. We urge you to delve into the material by mindfully but playfully exploring the activities to see what you discover about the concepts we present, but also about your own habits in relationship to these concepts. Chapter Six is about timing and the intimate role rhythm plays in movement, posture, and life itself. These chapters prepare you for Part Three: The Integrated Model, which weaves elements from the chapters in Part Two, rounding out the Framework into its aggregated whole.

Chapter 4

The Simple Model

The Language of Primary and Secondary

If you trace someone's spine with your hand, you will notice opposing curves: the neck region is concave, the thoracic region convex, the lumbar region concave, and the sacral region convex. The language we use to describe these curves relates to the initial spinal curve we were all born with, the Primary curves, and the curves that develop as we learn to sit and stand, the Secondary curves. As adults, these alternating curves provide mobility, strength, and resilience.

One of the things I realized . . . was that movement had to involve balancing the head with the tail. . . . It's this right up here [the suboccipital joint] always balancing with that right in there [the hip joints].

—Joan Murray, *Beginning from the Beginning*

For example, in tracing the spine that was just described, we can clarify this now by describing the neck/

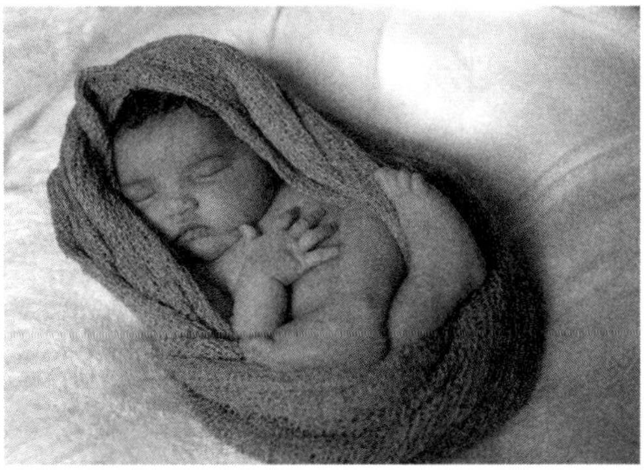

Overall Primary curve

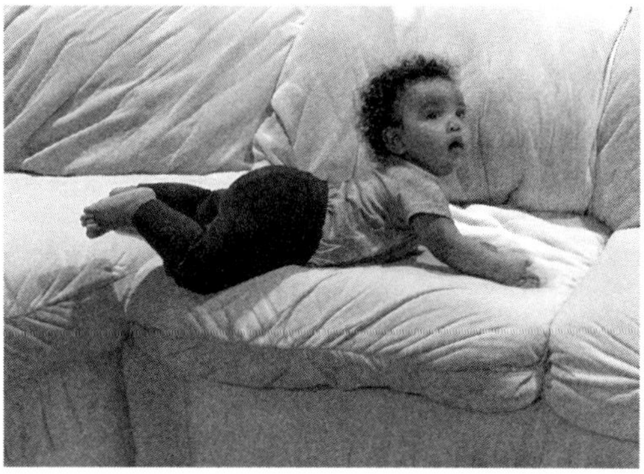

Secondary curves in cervical and lumbar spine

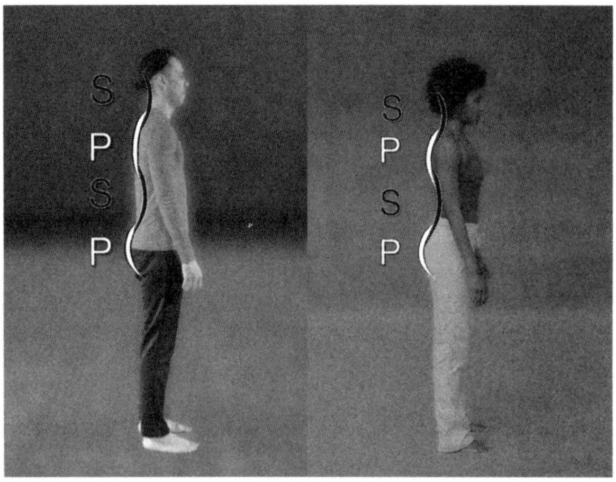

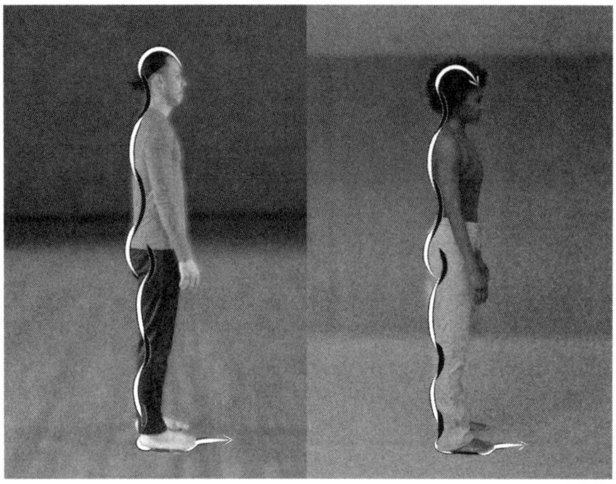

cervical region as a Secondary curve, the thoracic region as a Primary curve, the lumbar region as Secondary, and the sacrum as Primary.

We can expand this model to include the entire body structure. Additional primaries are: the top and the back of the head, the back of the upper legs (hamstrings), the calves, the heels, the balls of the feet, and the tips of the toes. Additional secondaries are: gluteals/outward rotators, the back of the knees, Achilles/back of ankles, arches of the feet, and under the toes.[1] We see these curves as generally balancing each other along the whole body. This provides a simple way to notice whether we interfere with this balance and the consequential disruption that may occur in the system. For example, if someone's spine tends toward a more overall Secondary approach, often the legs tend to balance this with more Primary than usual in the knee region, leading to a habitual hyperextension of the knees, or vice versa in terms of cause

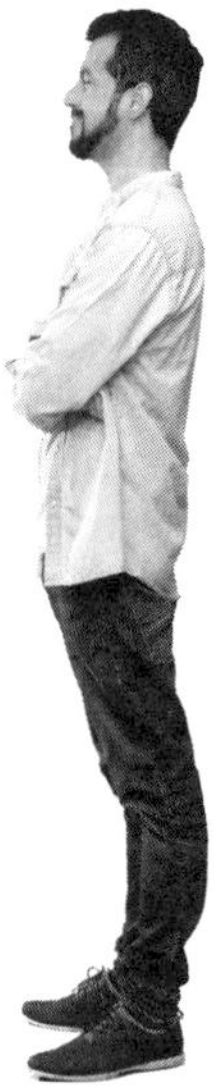

Hyperextended knees counterbalanced by flattening the spinal curves

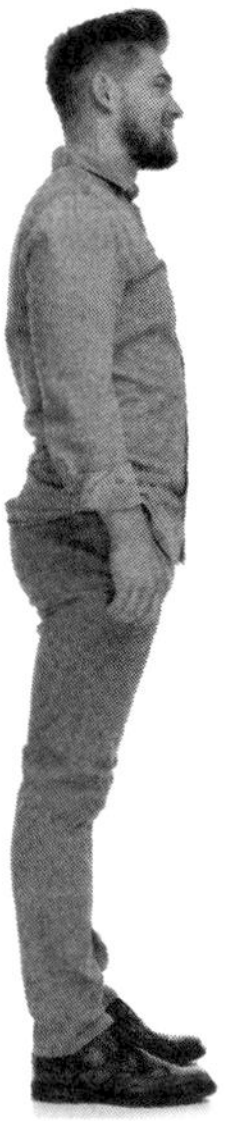

Over-engaged spinal Secondary curves, counterbalanced by hyperextended knees

and effect. Over-engaging or loading one curve of the system will be reflected in some way throughout the body.

> Something I thought was interesting about the reading was the statement that posture isn't really about holding a position but finding the right balance between the curves of your body that best support you and what you're doing. Almost all other conversations about posture I've been a part of center around holding a position, especially the times when teachers would tell me to "sit up straight." That direction doesn't give any instructions on how to get there. Thinking about the curves going all the way down the length of the body and not just the back really emphasizes how much the whole body is at work in this balancing, and how you shift between curves when you move. It's funny to me that the curves of the body and posture/alignment of them is so important to the way we develop and function in the world and can be the cause of many bodily issues or pains, yet we as a general society don't talk about it very much, at least in my experience. I feel like having more awareness of this earlier on in life would be beneficial.
>
> —Sydney Hagerman (Undergraduate dance student, University of Illinois)

Shape Versus Movement

Extending our model of the curves into movement, we would say that any movement toward flexion of the spine can be seen as going toward the Primary curve, and we would call that a Primary movement or activity. Likewise, moving into extension, or what we might call arching of the back, is a movement toward Secondary. For example, if you are sitting in a chair and you look down at the floor, allowing the whole body to adapt as you do so, you are moving toward Primary. If you look up and allow your whole body to participate in this movement, you are moving toward Secondary. Even though there are two opposing patterns in our structures, we are always moving toward one or the other, whether in the continuous act of breathing or in our various daily activities. In the Framework, Primary and Secondary are movements and directions, not simply curves or shapes.

The following linked video demonstrates Primary and Secondary movements with the help of straps to further indicate the movement's direction.

Video: Shape Versus Movement—Using Straps to Look Up and Down

Intent and Affinities

Intent is a key component in Primary and Secondary patterning. People act in accordance with a thought or intent, whether consciously or unconsciously. The Framework identifies the affinities for Primary and Secondary that encourage the best coordination. Affinities, as described in Chapter One, can be thought of as factors that belong to or go naturally with a movement or intention. In general,

Primary involves softening, folding, flexing, bending, curling in toward yourself. If you are standing, your gaze will go downward, your torso will curve forward, and your hips, knees, and ankles will bend. Movements related to Primary include the toddler squatting to play, bending forward to pick something up off the floor, and the gymnast performing a forward somersault.

Secondary involves the opposite: extending, reaching, arching, going out into the world. If you are standing, your gaze will go upward, your back will tend to arch, your hips will extend, knees lengthen, and ankles thrust away from the earth. Movements related to Secondary include the toddler reaching to be picked up, going up on tiptoes to reach for a cup out of the cupboard, and the diver arching before going into the water. Both Primary and Secondary movements take place in the sagittal plane and are generally homologous/symmetrical.

At times, a shape may seem to indicate one curve, but the activity is, in fact, the opposite. Take the example of a skydiver falling through the air, arms and legs outstretched in what looks like Secondary. But the activity here is actually Primary, because the sky diver is pushing down against the current of air that is coming up to meet his body. Or you might be in a Primary curve, for example, in a curved position seated on a chair with your head resting on a desk in front of you, eyes closed. The moment you think about looking up and out and open your eyes, you are already going toward Secondary. So it is important not to focus on the shape the body is making, but rather to see the movement and the forces that either facilitate or oppose it.

Affinities of Participation of Limbs in Primary and Secondary

MOVEMENT EXPLORATION 4.1:
FULL BODY PRIMARY AND SECONDARY

You can experience the overall affinities of the arms and legs, first by lying prone on a soft surface (massage table, carpet), with your forehead down on the surface, and the arms down by your sides. Allow your arms to rotate inward, so that the palms are facing

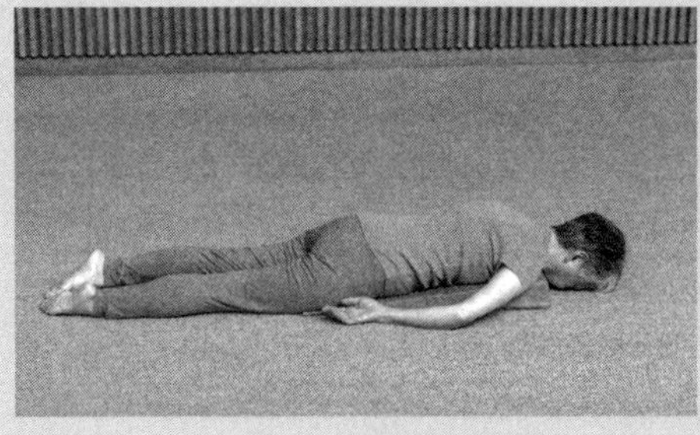

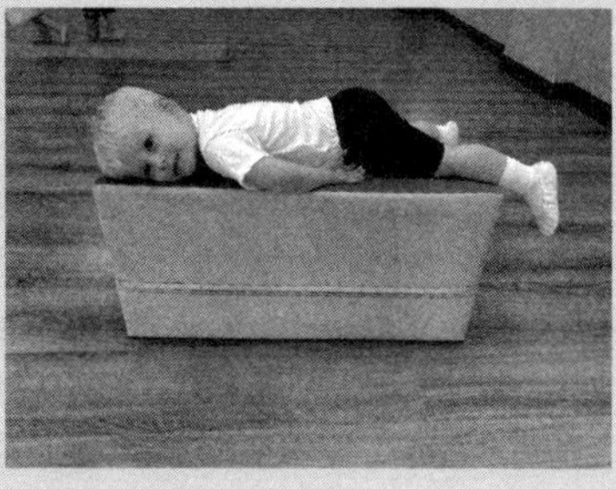

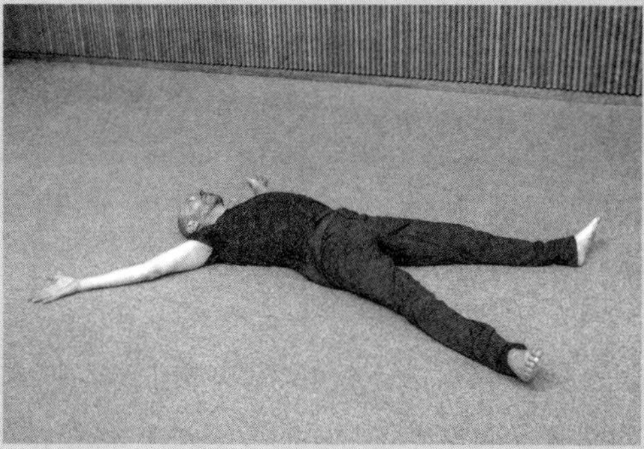

upward, and allow the legs to turn in (toes in toward the midline). Let your whole back soften and feel a sense of width. This is a full-body Primary. Make sure you are not trying to press your pelvis down toward the floor. If it is uncomfortable to keep your forehead down, you can turn your head and lie on your cheek.

Now roll over to your back. Allow the legs to turn out, let the arms be turned out, palms up, and be sure you are not pushing your lower back down toward the floor, but allow the secondary curve of the lumbar to be present. This is a full-body Secondary.

Now come to a standing position and look down toward your sternum, and continue that direction of the curve of the back, while letting your hips/knees/ankles bend. At the same time, let your arms rotate inward. Reverse this by coming up to look up to the ceiling, straightening your legs, and allowing your arms to turn out.

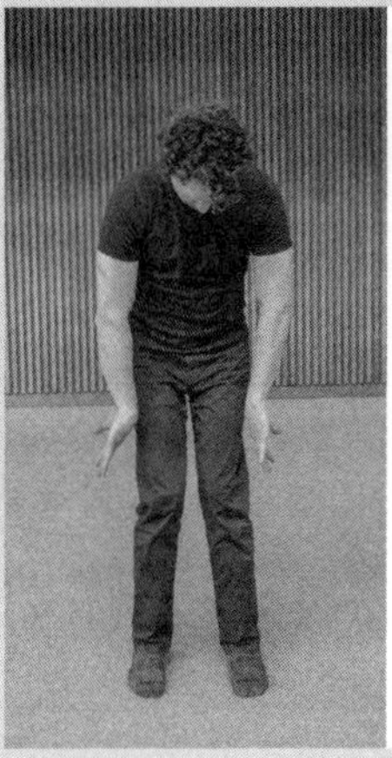

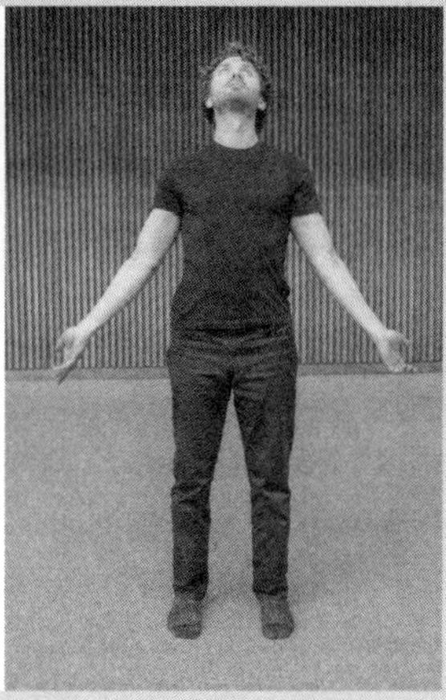

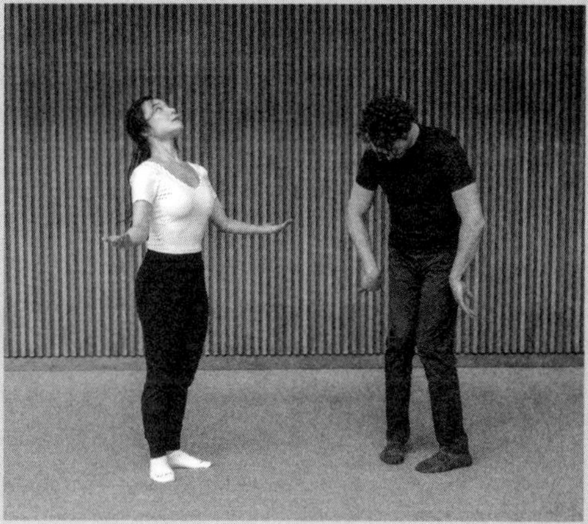

This week we continued to explore different variations of the primary and secondary curves. I began to be more aware of how the shoulder blades are related to the motion of the spine. When we stood and did our primary curve, Professor Nettl-Fiol gave us the hint to rotate our arms inwards even more deliberately. This didn't come very naturally to me at first, as it did in the lying-down position. But as soon as I found the way to do it, there was a sudden relaxation of the muscles surrounding the shoulder blades, involving the back, ribs, and neck. I could literally visualize the arch of my back becoming smoother. There was an expansion of my upper back towards the ceiling, and breathing felt easier as well. As I transferred to secondary curve, the shoulder blades felt so much more alive, as they naturally made a big circle turning outwards, opening up like flower petals.

—Yuemeng Li, Music graduate student, University of Illinois

Here we have explored the basic affinities of the arms and legs in relation to Primary and Secondary, where the limbs turn in as part of the Primary pattern and turn out as part of the Secondary pattern. Next, we will look at supporting the intended activities of the arms or legs with the proper engagement of the back. To explore this, try the following movement exercise:

MOVEMENT EXPLORATION 4.2: AFFINITY FOR ARMS IN SECONDARY

Lie on the floor in a prone position, with elbows bent, forearms on the floor, and thumbs near the mouth. This is akin to a baby during "tummy time." You are basically in a Primary. Now, have an intention of wanting to see or smell something in front of you. Look up toward it, and as a baby might do, see if your body responds by: 1) a pull of the forearms from the hands to the elbows, in an effort to help you with your wish to go forward, and 2) an engagement of turning out in the legs. These would both be affinities for Secondary, so that the whole of you is engaged in the desire to go forward.

Notice whether you really are allowing your arms to participate. If you are not engaging your hands and forearms as you look up, you may find that you are overusing your neck. If you feel caught, it may be due to an under-engagement of the arms, an undue tightening of the abdominals, or other factors that could be interfering with the overall intention to go forward.

If you have a partner to work with, try this variation to see whether you are, in fact, allowing the arms to participate.

MOVEMENT EXPLORATION 4.3: PARTNER EXPLORATION OF ARMS IN LOOKING UP

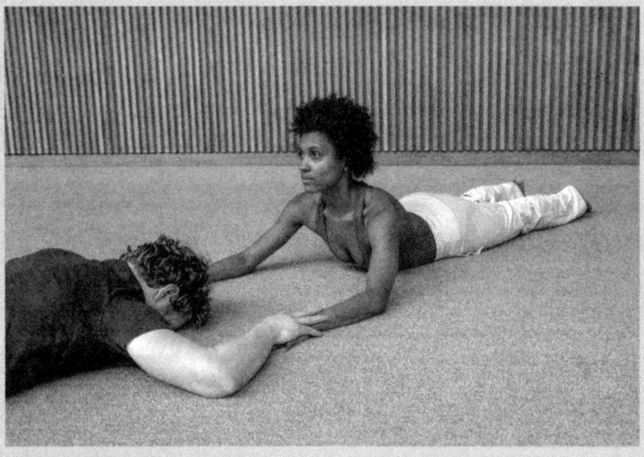

Both partners lie prone on the floor, heads toward each other, and arms forward on the floor with elbows bent, palms down. Partner (A), put your hands on top of Partner (B)'s forearms, and close your eyes so that you will be able to feel what happens to Partner (B)'s arms. Partner (B), look forward and up, as in the previous Movement Exploration. Partner (A), see if you can say (without looking) when Partner (B) is looking up and when she has put her head back down. Discuss what you notice. Then switch roles.

This exploration clearly illustrates the consequential engagement of the arms that occurs automatically if one does not interfere with the movement's sequencing.

MOVEMENT EXPLORATION 4.4: AFFINITY FOR ARMS IN PRIMARY

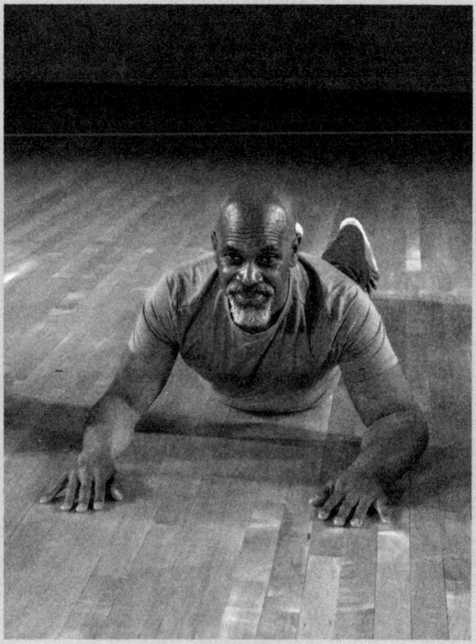

Begin on hands and knees, like a baby about to crawl. Look forward toward something that interests you (you are in Secondary). Now give up that interest and push yourself back onto your haunches. This is a Primary. The arm affinity for Primary is a push.

Go back to your belly (prone) and look up, taking the weight also on your forearms, like a baby looking up, with the head free to look around. Tuck your toes under and rock forward and backward. Notice the subtle alternation of Primary and Secondary that occurs even in this small movement. When you rock forward, the arms pull and ankles plantar flex, while the toes push. When you rock backward, the arms push and the ankles dorsiflex.

Notice the kinetic chain of movement in this rocking action. Do you find a holding place, or a place that is caught or blocked, such that the rocking stops or is unable to pass through the whole body? If so, this gives you information about possible holding patterns.

MOVEMENT EXPLORATION 4.5: SWINGING ARMS BACK AND FORTH

Begin in a standing position and then lift your arms to the front. This action would best be supported by Primary, where your back is not necessarily going into an obvious curve, but it is wide and strong, countering the movement of the arms going forward by staying back and away from the fingertips. From there, if you swing your arms down and to the back, the whole spine can change, by allowing a slight Secondary activity, letting the gaze go upward slightly, the legs thrusting away from the floor, and the back releasing from the Primary into more length. If you swing your arms back and forth with these things in mind, you will see how much adaptation of the whole self can occur during this movement.

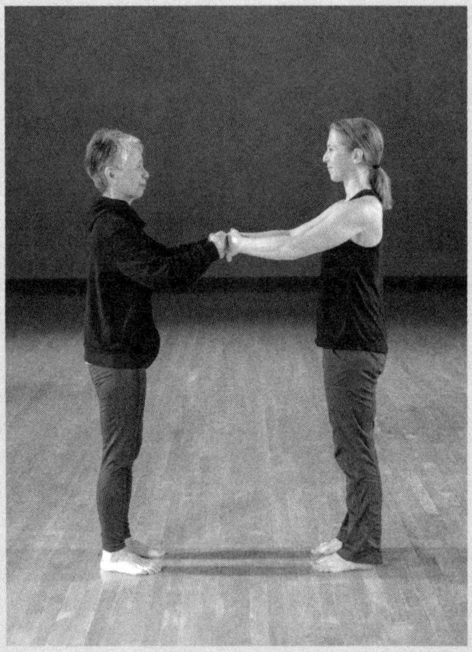

MOVEMENT EXPLORATION 4.6: PRIMARY PUSH WITH ARMS

You can do this movement exploration with a partner or a wall. Stand across from your partner and both of you lift your arms toward each other, ending with touching the backs of your hands together. Elbows should be a little bit bent, so your arms are rounded. If you are using a wall, touch the wall with the backs of your hands. Be sure you are standing close enough to each other that you are balanced on your feet, with your bodies vertical. Give a little bit of a push to each other, and allow your knees, ankles, and hips to bend slightly as you push. Let your backs support the movement in a Primary.

Things to notice:

- Do you have a tendency to round your back?
- Are your shoulders shrugging up?
- Are you aware of your *whole* back, or only a part?

If you are working with a partner, you can try a variation of this exercise, where one partner walks forward, causing the other partner to walk backward. Notice that both partners must maintain the Primary Engagement in their backs for this movement to be successful. If one partner releases the back into Secondary, the other partner will feel it immediately, and the smooth walking will be disrupted. You can play with shifting the lead, so that the other partner leads by walking forward.

Video: Ballroom Walking Forward and Back with Your Hands Touching and Your Back in Primary

In many movement forms requiring both defensive and offensive maneuvers, such as martial arts practices, pushing with the back of the hands and wrists is a familiar practice or physical experience. The Primary push that sends the distal ends of the arms farther away from the back also facilitates strength—think of boxing or punching with the knuckles as a strong, overall Primary *push*. In the Dart Procedures, as the mover "devolves" through anthropoidal postures, the torso comes up and away from knuckles that are extended to the seat of a chair or the floor in the deepest expressions of full-body Primary. This echoes the way primates ambulate by pushing themselves away from the ground with their knuckles.

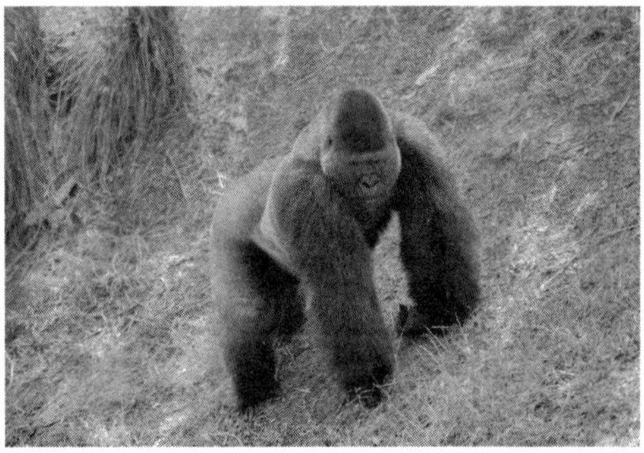

MOVEMENT EXPLORATION 4.7: SECONDARY PULL WITH ARMS

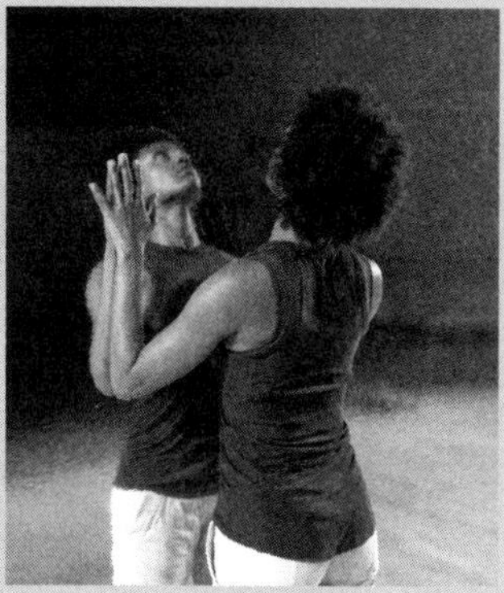

Face your partner again, in a slight knee bend, and raise your arms toward each other, but this time, switch the position of your hands so that your fingers hold on to each other's. Now both of you give a little pull against each other and look up slightly, bringing yourselves up from the bent knee position, all the way onto toes. This is a Secondary activity.

If you are using the wall instead of a partner, get close enough to the wall so that you can put your palms and lower arms against it. Look up as if you want to climb up the wall, and pull yourself, so that you go up onto your toes.

Again, we are exploring the affinities of Primary and Secondary in these activities.

Reset

We discussed the term Reset in Chapter Three. It is quite applicable and easy to understand in relation to Primary and Secondary, in that you can Engage in Primary and Reset from it or Engage in Secondary and Reset from it. Resetting from one inevitably takes you toward the other. The simplest way to illustrate this is with movement of the hand and fingers. If you make a tight fist, you are Engaging in Primary. If you simply release that Engagement, you are going toward Secondary, even though your hand is still a little bit curved. But in letting go of the Engagement, you Reset in the opposite direction. Now if you fully extend your hand, stretching your fingers out as far as you can, you are moving into Secondary. If you let go of that Engagement, you are Resetting toward Primary.[2] Resetting is most easily experienced if you allow yourself to fully Engage in the action that precedes it.

MOVEMENT EXPLORATION 4.8: PRIMARY RESET IN A CHAIR

Sit in a chair, with your feet on the floor and lower legs perpendicular to the floor, and your hands on your thighs. From there, look down toward your sternum and allow the rest of the body to respond to this Primary inclination, by allowing the back ribs to soften and the spine to soften and curve. Continue rolling forward as far as is comfortable. Now imagine there is something that smells good out in front of you. Begin to look up to see what that smell is, and as you do so, allow your arms to help you by holding on to your knees, and allowing a slight pull of your hands on your knees. Really engage in this activity of looking out and smelling something good way out in front as you start to come up. When you get about halfway up to sitting, just give up the whole idea, letting yourself Reset to return to sitting upright again. You will be in the same general position as when you started, but it will be a renewed, or refreshed, place.

Video: Primary Reset in a Chair

MOVEMENT EXPLORATION 4.9: PRIMARY RESET ON A BED

Sit on a bed, a couch, or a soft mat, with your knees bent and feet flat on the floor. You can hold on to your lower legs if that is comfortable, or put your hands on the floor next to you to help support yourself. Now look up toward the ceiling, really letting yourself reach your whole self upward. Make sure you are aiming to go up, not dropping your head back. When you feel you have extended as fully as you can, let yourself Reset by giving up the upward intention, nodding the head forward, and falling back toward the bed, ending in an overall Primary.

Video: Primary Reset on a Bed

In these two movement explorations, it is important to ascertain whether you were able to let go of the Engagement to allow the Reset to occur, or whether you were actively Engaging in the opposite activity. Resetting is not about *doing the contrasting action* but about *undoing the previous one.* This letting go can be more challenging than you might think, as we often are habitually attached to *doing,* so that *non-doing* may seem lazy or inaccessible.

Interferences

Using the lens of Primary and Secondary allows us to observe when we are interfering, whether it is through habit or through misunderstanding the intent of the movement. Keeping the affinities in mind, if someone is getting ready to sit in a chair, which we would identify as a Primary activity, and she over-engages the neck by pulling the head back and down in preparation, we could describe this as an inappropriate overuse of Secondary. The reverse of this would be someone who over-engages Primary by contracting the abdominals, or "crunching" the spine when getting ready to stand up.

Another example is someone looking down but not allowing the back and hips and knees to bend, so that all the flexion occurs in the neck and upper back. The Primary then becomes isolated in the head/neck area, while the rest of the body is Engaging in Secondary. Or we might see someone sitting in a slumped position in a chair, looking up at a person who is talking to them, but not allowing their whole body to extend and participate in the direction of their gaze. Here the Secondary gets isolated in the head and neck, while the rest of the body stays in Primary. You can imagine that this would be very tiring on the head/neck/shoulder area. Knowing the affinities gives you tools for discovering where you might be interfering habitually without realizing it.

Of course, one does not necessarily always have to align movement with the affinities. Maybe you feel like stretching your hamstrings and keeping your knees straight when bending over. Maybe you want to Engage in each alternating activity rather than finding the opportunities to Reset, if you are doing strength training, for example. But these should be *conscious choices* rather than unconscious habitual patterns.

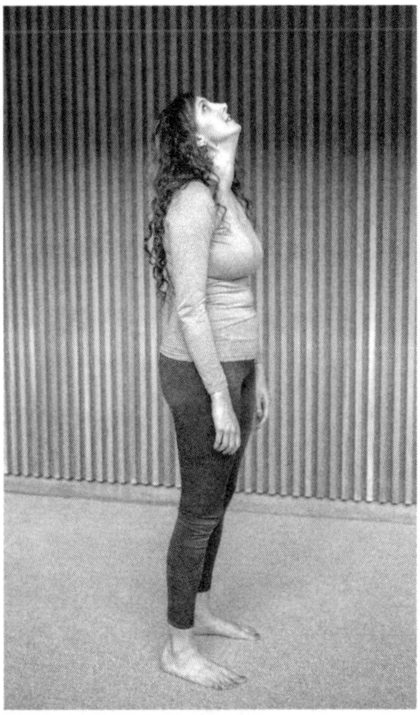
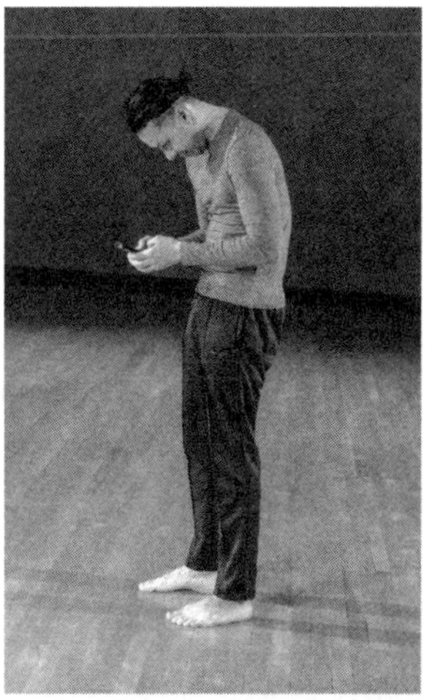

Examples of common interferences

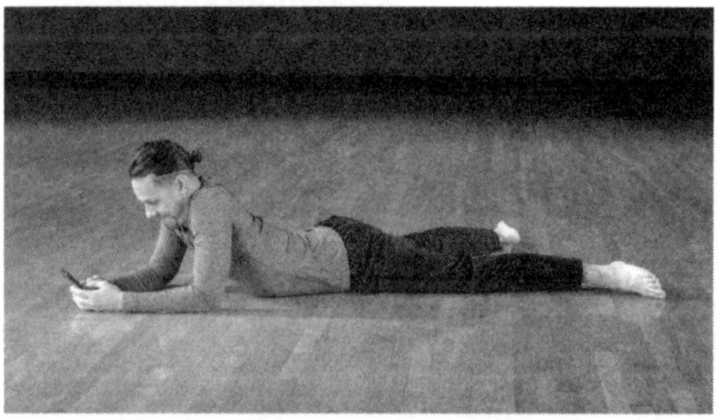
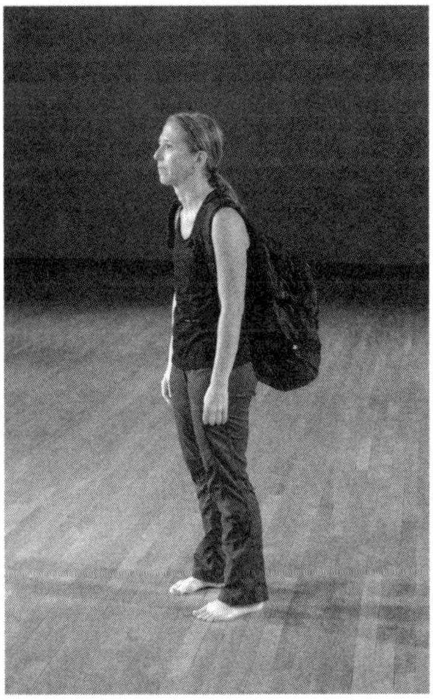
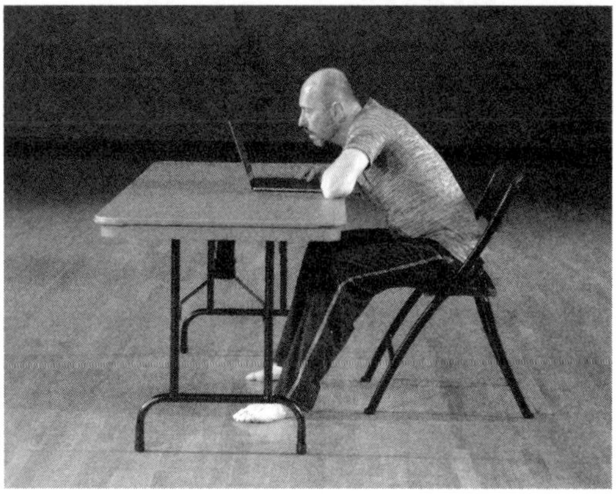

The Lively Interplay

There is a constant interaction between Primary and Secondary, and between Engagement and Reset. These movements can occur on a big scale or simply in thought. As you move, you want to be able to adjust appropriately to the action, even on a subtle level. And you want to be available for these adjustments to occur, not locked or fixed in a certain pattern. Let's say you go to shake hands with someone. That may be an overall Secondary activity, as you are interested in the person in front of you and want to extend yourself toward them. But then after that, do you allow yourself to Reset out of this when you have finished greeting them? Knowing your own tendencies in relation to Primary and Secondary is useful for recognizing when these kinds of situations occur.

On a more subtle level, we could equate Secondary with the idea of lengthening and Primary with the idea of widening. In the Alexander Technique, we talk about allowing the lengthening and widening of the back to occur. At times, we may want to emphasize one more than the other, depending on the activity, and depending on our own individual habit or preference. But it is important to allow for the interplay between the two ideas. When both are present and operating in tandem, we find integration.

MOVEMENT EXPLORATION 4.10: THINKING TOWARD PRIMARY AND SECONDARY

Stand and put the palm of one hand on the top of your head, and the back of your hand somewhere on your mid-back. First, in an exaggerated manner, reach your head up to your hand. Notice that your back probably narrowed and went away from your back hand. Now release that and instead, push your back into your back hand. Notice that your head probably lowered from your top hand.

Now, instead of "doing" these movements in an exaggerated way, try simply thinking of these directions. First, *just think* about your head going toward your top hand. Then, *just think* about your back going toward your back hand. Now see if you can think both at the same time.

If you have a partner, it is possible to do this exploration with the partner's hands on you rather than having your own hands on yourself. Your partner also may be able to notice what you are doing and thinking, and then give you feedback.

Things to notice:

- Is your breath affected by any of the "doing"?
- Is there a difference in breath between really trying to *do* the directions, compared to primarily *thinking* the directions?

Summary

The applications of this portion of the Framework are endless. Primary and Secondary Engagements and Resets form the building blocks for the rest of the Framework, creating a dynamic reciprocity in the body. Our goal is to bring awareness to this underlying system so that we can regain control of a more balanced, adaptable ongoing exchange in the body overall. We wish to match our intentions with the supporting activity of Primary or Secondary, and to be able to notice when intent conflicts with our habitual actions or movement patterns.

Applications of Primary and Secondary to Breastfeeding

Claire Happel Ashe

When my son was born, the lactation consultant described a breastfeeding position called the "laid back" or "natural" position. It is a position inspired by mammalian feeding in general, and it lets the baby and gravity (rather than the mother) do a lot of the work, which attracted me! It also emphasizes the positioning of the mother first, then the baby, then the breast, which reminded me of teaching the Alexander Technique, in which we prioritize our own use as we put a hand on a student to help them be aware of theirs. By positioning the mother in a comfortable position in the chair before supporting her breast, I also felt it emphasized the mother's whole self first, rather than narrowing down myopically to the point of contact where the baby is feeding.

The mother arranges herself in a very Primary position in a chair—hips forward, shoulders and head resting on the couch—and the baby lies skin-to-skin on the mother's belly. In that way, the torso holds the weight of the baby instead of the arms. The tactile feedback on the baby's chest and abdomen, the bottoms of his feet, and the insides of his knees against the mother's torso stimulates the baby in a reflexive way to start lifting his head and reaching his mouth. I thought, "Wow! How amazing that this tactile contact is reflexively inspiring into a full secondary curve to reach for food." Just as we think of external rotation of the legs and upward thrust in ballet as an affinity of Secondary, this primal reflex from tactile contact brought him into a strong secondary curve to get what he needed to survive. It was beautiful and one of the most helpful pieces of advice I got as a new mother. My son and I still use this position one year in!

Applications of Primary and Secondary in Lower Extremity Loss

Physical Therapist Maryhelen Wesner

I like to think that I'm pretty good at sitting. I bet you do too. But for some, it's not so easy. Hi. I'm a physical therapist, and I've been working with people with lower extremity limb loss for the past fifteen years. When beginning to teach a person to use their new prosthetic legs, one of the first physical therapy sessions includes learning to stand up and sit down. This becomes more difficult if two legs have been amputated rather than one, and it is even further complicated by amputations above the knee. I'd like to tell you about a time when I used my understanding of Framework for Integration to inform my physical therapy practice for an individual with bilateral transfemoral amputations.

"James" sustained amputations to both legs, above the knee. He is a young adult, otherwise healthy, and has excellent, well-fitting prosthetic legs with microprocessor knees. Basically, if prosthetic legs were cars, these would be luxury class. And yet sitting down was a huge challenge for him. While there really is no official physical therapy recipe for teaching someone to sit down, there are verbal and physical cues that I have found to be helpful to assist the person to use the prostheses' full potential. Unfortunately, in this case, nothing seemed to work. As he hammered away at this skill, I identified that as his effort and frustration grew, so did his Secondary posture. Instead of being able to ride the knees down, as they are programmed to do, he would bend his upper body forward and then fall back in the chair. PLOP. The harder he tried, the harder he landed.

After many unsuccessful tries, I let him know that while I appreciated his hard work, I wanted this to be gentler. I put my hand on his back, asked him to take a moment to soften his posture (towards Primary), and to rest down into the chair. And with that, for the very first time since before his accident, he was able to sit with ease and control. Honestly, it was a breakthrough moment for us both.

NOTES

1. We have expanded Thomas Myers's initial description of the "waves of the spine" from his 2001 publication, *Anatomy Trains* (88–89).
2. Allyna Steinberg first suggested this example of making a fist when attending one of our workshops.

Chapter 5

The Complex Model

Spiral

> **Man suspends the remainder of his body from his head and spine. He swings his body from his head by means of two spirally arranged but interwoven sheets of voluntary musculature in exactly the same manner that his fishy and amphibian forefathers swung their bodies from their heads.**
>
> **—Raymond Dart, "Voluntary Musculature in the Human Body: The Double-Spiral Arrangement," from *Skill and Poise***

The Simple Model looks at movements and curves in the sagittal plane—forward and backward motions with flexion and extension. The Complex Model builds on this by addressing our double-spiral musculature, as first described by Raymond Dart in his 1950 article, "Voluntary Musculature of the Human Body: The Double-Spiral Arrangement," reflecting the human body's intricate and three-dimensional design. If you look at a human skeleton, you may notice that not even one bone in the body is absolutely straight! We are built with a series of spirals, from the double helix structures of our DNA to the way our muscles evolved from a series of spiral sheets that wrap around the body during fetal development (Dart 1996, 67–70). These sheets develop into differentiated muscle groups in the body as it matures from fetus to newborn, and newborn to child. But the underlying design can be seen in the connectivities within the musculofascial system (Myers 2001).

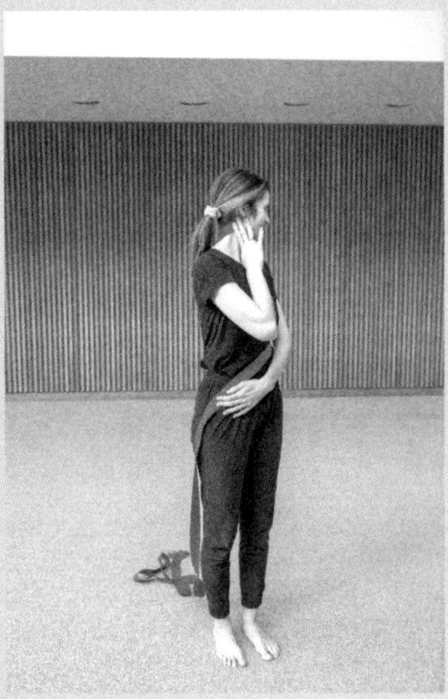

MOVEMENT EXPLORATION 5.1:
BANDS TO ILLUSTRATE SIMPLE SPIRAL

Using a yoga strap or a TheraBand, hold one end just at the back of the right ear (mastoid process). Wrap the strap going behind the neck, downward and to the left, then around the ribs, following their angle to travel to the front of the body, across the midline, to attach to the right hip bone (anterior superior iliac spine—ASIS). This represents one spiral line that catches the splenius, rhomboids, intercostals, external and internal obliques. If you turn your head to the right, you are shortening this spiral (you will feel the slackening of the strap). If you turn your head left, you are lengthening this spiral (you will feel the tension of the strap). Notice that your head is connected to the same hip, but through a line that wraps around the body, rather than linearly from point to point.

In the Framework, we see the double-spiral as a complex diagonal interweaving of Primary and Secondary curves throughout the body, so that a movement of any part affects the movement of the whole.

Identifying Primary and Secondary Inside the Spiral

MOVEMENT EXPLORATION 5.2:
IDENTIFYING PRIMARY AND SECONDARY IN A CHAIR, SPIRALING

If you are sitting in a chair, you can think of a relationship between your right shoulder and your left hip, and vice versa. Turn and look around to your right to see someone or something behind you, allowing your weight to shift from being evenly on two hips to having more weight on your right hip. You can notice that the front of your left shoulder gets closer to the front of your right hip (a Primary relationship), while the front of your right shoulder gets farther away from the front of your left hip (a Secondary relationship). Allow the left hip to lead you back to center so you are again balanced on both hips. To enhance the experience of the Primary aspect of this spiral, you can try the sequence again, but this time, place the left hand on the front of the right hip, and as you turn to look to the right, let the left hand continue sliding toward the back of the right hip as you go. This helps your left shoulder girdle participate more in the Primary activity of the spiral.

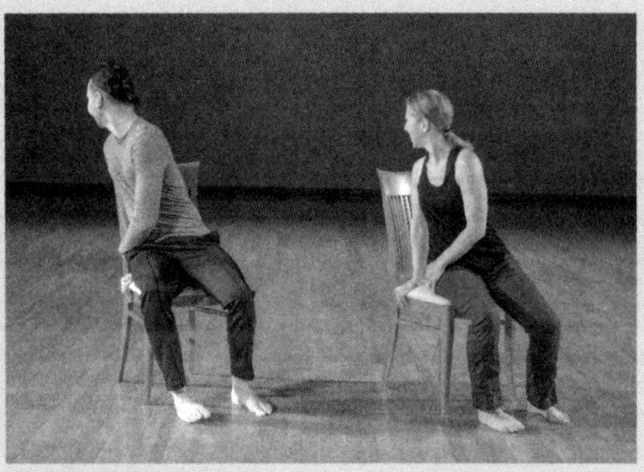

Spiraling in the chair was also extremely impactful for me due to the Reset that takes place at the end. While exploring the exercise I found that my habit on the Reset was to collapse my spine instead of keeping the length that is created during the exercise.
—Anthony DeGregorio, Theatre graduate student, University of Illinois

You also might notice whether you allowed the legs to change while you performed this spiral. In our definition of a spiral, there is always a weight shift, and subsequently, the legs will also adjust to the spiraling activity. If you turn to the right as above, the right ankle will supinate and the left ankle will pronate if you allow them to do so.

Things to notice:

- As you spiral to the right, do you notice any resistance in the left shoulder? Does it want to stay open? Notice that crossing the left hand to right hip will help with this habit/interference.
- Do it on the other side. Did you notice different habits?

We see here that the Primary and Secondary curves actually cross as we spiral, following one trajectory of the double-spiral around the body in a Primary (the spiral that shortens), while the Secondary lengthens. The Primary spiral provides support while the Secondary spiral promotes length, encouraging movement into space.

We can observe this in a baby who rolls from his belly to his back. As he turns to look over the right shoulder, there is a Secondary curve from the right shoulder to the left hip, counterbalanced by the Primary curve from the left shoulder to the right hip. In this example, the right leg will tend to bend and rotate out, while the left leg will tend to straighten and rotate in. Ultimately, this spiral initiation will result in the baby rolling onto his back—a Reset.

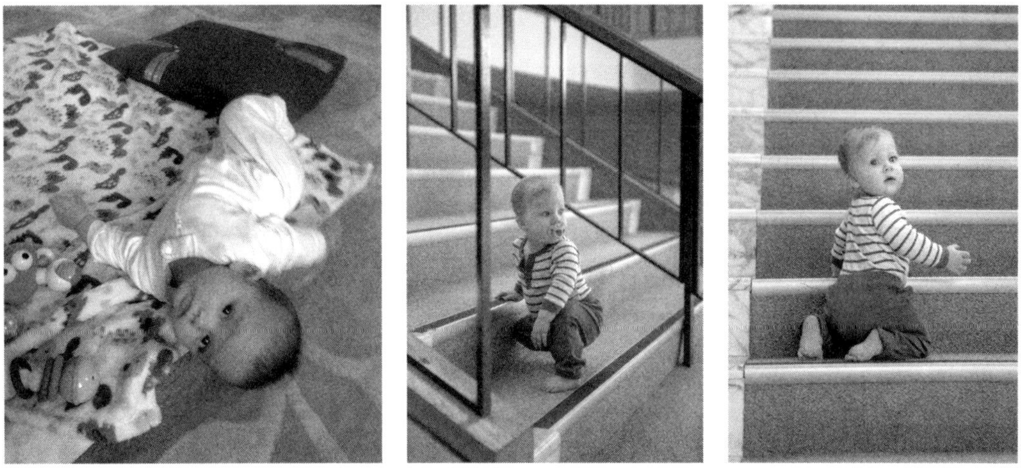

MOVEMENT EXPLORATION 5.3:
SPIRAL ROLL AND RESET

Try this for yourself! Lying on your belly, look to your right and continue looking around, as if you want to see something behind you. Allow your weight to shift toward your left hip as you continue to look. While doing so, you can add a slight push against the ground with your right hand, and you can extend your left arm overhead along the floor. On the way to rolling over, notice whether your right knee bends and the leg turns out, while the left leg straightens. Once you go so far that you have no choice but to roll onto your back, experience the Reset of that action.

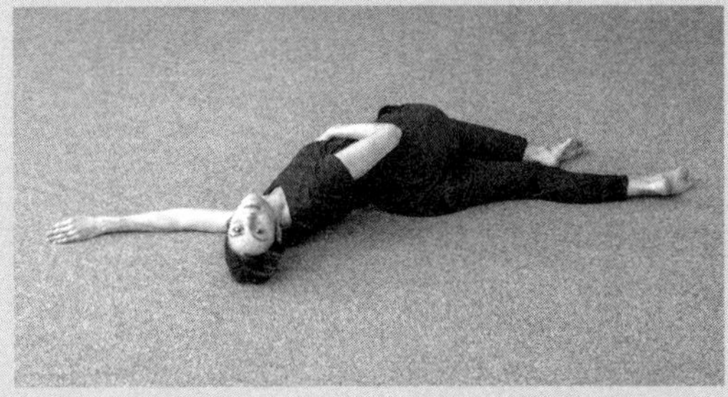

In this movement exploration, there are many things to notice.

- Did you find that looking around led to a weight shift? If not, can you identify what was holding on to prevent this from happening?
- Did your right hip try to lead the movement? If so, see if you can let it wait until the inevitable time when it needs to go with the rolling.
- Did you tend to keep much of your back in Secondary, or could you find the crossing of the Primary and Secondary?
- Were you able to find the oppositional bending of one knee and straightening of the other?
- Were you able to Reset for the roll to complete, or did you control it?

Now we will explore the opposite: Arching to roll from the back to the front.

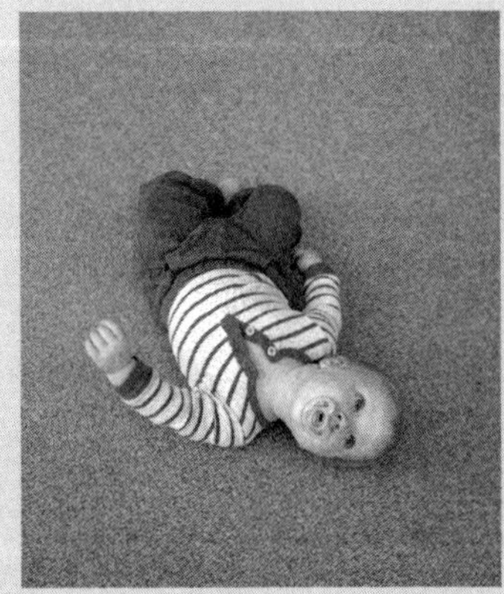

MOVEMENT EXPLORATION 5.4:
ROLLING FROM THE BACK TO THE FRONT

Lying on your back, with both arms out to your sides, imagine there is something enticing you to look around behind you and to your right. You might want to imagine yourself as a baby wanting desperately to roll over! As you turn your head to the right, shift your weight onto your right hip and arch your back. As you allow for the stretch of the left side of the neck to occur, also notice that from your left shoulder to your right hip is a Primary relationship, while your right shoulder to your left hip is Secondary. Make sure you are not stiffening your legs. Now allow your right arm to slide overhead as you continue this spiral motion to flip over to your belly. Again, this inevitable flip is a Reset, or a result of the spiral.

Video: Rolling from the Back to the Front

In both these examples, the spiral is initiated by the head/sensory stimuli (wanting to see, smell, hear something), and the body follows sequentially. In this type of spiral movement, the Secondary spiral is dominant in leading the movement into space, while the Primary spiral is supportive, giving connectivity to the body as it engages in the movement.

MOVEMENT EXPLORATION 5.5: SPIRALING TO STANDING

This movement exploration offers another example where the head leads the body into a spiral that launches the body into action. Begin by sitting in a chair. Imagine that someone behind you calls your name. Look around to the right, allowing the spiral to shift your weight to your right hip and sequentially follow your head to stand up. In other words, let the head direction lead you to standing. (Try this to your left as well and see which side might be your preference.)

Video: Spiraling to Standing

Things to notice:

- How could the patterning and sequencing in this movement exploration make everyday activities easier?
- Can you notice that one leg moves more toward inward rotation and the other toward outward?

A useful application of this movement exploration is getting out of a car. You can find an ease in the motion by looking and immediately transferring the weight to one side to lead you up and out of the car.

> The most AHA moment for me was the standing from a spiral. Leading with the intention and allowing the head to lead my spine to a standing position through my spirals was absolutely mind-blowing, and gave my legs the greatest gift of ease. I've never felt so free, light, and buoyant. I also absolutely loved being able to have a moment of realization about how our spine is supported in a three-dimensional way as opposed to it just being flat ridged layers of two-dimensional muscle. It makes so much sense, and is a wonderful gift of knowledge about myself.
>
> —Anthony DeGregorio, Theatre graduate student, University of Illinois

Spiraling stimulates a weight shift either toward something or away, depending on the context. Movement Exploration 5.5 directed you to shift in the direction of the spiral. But, for example, if you're sitting in a chair and look to your right, you could also choose to shift your weight to your left hip. Maybe you are in your office,

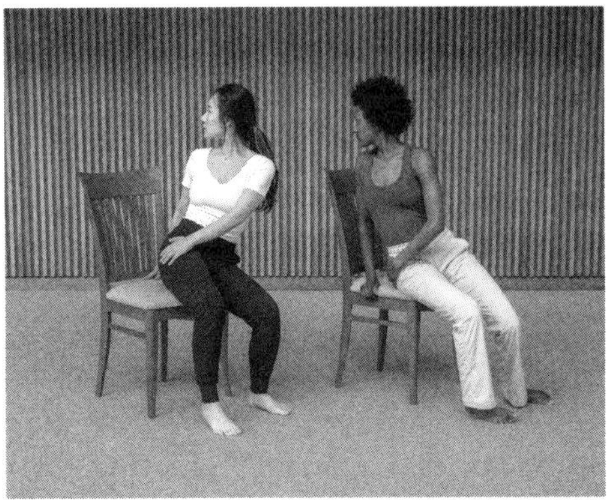

and someone comes and stands at your right side to speak to you. You could turn your head toward them but shift your weight away to give yourself more space and enable you to look at them more easily. This type of weight shift is appropriate in plenty of situations. That being said, we propose that it is not the *direction* of the weight shift that is important, but that you are allowing your weight to shift one way or the other, as this is an integral aspect of spiraling.

Counterspirals (One Against the Other)

The previous examples employ the sequential flow or continuity and follow-through of the spiral in motion. The next spiral pattern we will discuss is the counterspiral: the interlocking of two spirals, where part of the body spirals in one direction, countered by another part spiraling in the opposite direction.

MOVEMENT EXPLORATION 5.6: COUNTERSPIRAL IN A CHAIR

Sitting in a chair, turn your head to look behind you to your right, allowing a spiral to occur so that your torso follows, the weight shifts to the right, your left hand traces your right leg to end up on the outside of your right thigh, and your legs adapt to this spiral as well. Now, maintaining this spiral, look around toward the left shoulder so that you have one spiral opposing the other. An alternative pathway is to look up toward the ceiling, encouraging a bit of lengthening before looking around to the left shoulder. In either case, now let your gaze lower slightly toward your left shoulder. Notice that there is a Primary relationship between your left cheek and your left shoulder. In this dynamic position, you are experiencing two opposing spirals in the body. Now just let go of these spirals to Reset, and you will unwind back to center.

Video: Counterspiral in a Chair

One spiral working antagonistically against another promotes connectivity. This type of counterspiral activity provides a coil, where the unwinding of both spirals supplies power without having to overwork. We often liken this coiling action to the spring in a pogo stick or an old-fashioned bed coil; when pressure is loaded into the coil and then released, the coil simply rebounds. The tennis serve illustrates the windup into one spiral that releases into the other. When we hit a baseball with a bat, throw a ball, or launch the body forward in skating on the ice, we are using the two opposing spirals in the body. Practically everything we do involves spiraling. When we walk, we switch from one spiral to another, made possible by our ability to Reset in between.

MOVEMENT EXPLORATION 5.7: WALKING

Explore walking by paying attention to the spirals that exchange as you step from one foot to the other. As you step forward on the right foot, notice the Primary spiral that can occur between the left shoulder and the right hip, and the Secondary spiral between the right shoulder and left hip. Think about the image of slightly crumpling the Primary spiral (like an accordion) to exaggerate the Engagement of Primary. Then allow that crumpling activity to Reset, which propels you up and forward to shift weight onto your left foot, where you will switch the spirals so that the Primary spiral is now from your right shoulder to your left hip, while the Secondary is from your left shoulder to your right hip. You are Resetting from one spiral to the next as you walk. You can try this in a more exaggerated way to get a feeling for the experience of the spirals and Resets, and then after that, you can try this in a more subtle way. The arms participate by swinging in opposition to the stepping and, in fact, are an extension of the spirals.

Video: Walking

Notice that your head maintains its forward focus while the body spirals underneath, creating a counterspiral. Notice also that there is an inherent rhythm or timing associated with the spirals that facilitates the spring, or the Reset involved in the action.

Twist

In the Framework, we insist spirals necessarily include weight shifting. What happens when we want to keep the pelvis stable while turning the upper body in a spiral? We differentiate this type of movement from a spiral, calling it a twist, where the base stays fixed as the free end rotates. So in a sense, it could be thought of as a counterspiral.

MOVEMENT EXPLORATION 5.8: TWISTING

Stand with the feet underneath the hip joints. Think of the two hip bones (anterior superior iliac spines, or ASIS) as headlights (this image is commonly used in dance training). Keep your headlights pointing forward as you turn your head and upper body to the right. Reset and return to center.

Now try this movement again, but instead of headlights, consider what happens when you let your weight shift very slightly to the left, counter-spiraling the pelvis to the left as the upper body spirals to the right. Then Reset and go back to center.

Now try this movement once again, but just *think* of the lower body as following this spiral, allowing your weight to shift very slightly to the right, even though it doesn't really shift in space.

Which of these three alternatives felt more dynamic and active, with less strain? There are many ways to do a movement. We propose the last two options provide more opportunity for resilience and put less pressure on the lower back and the joints overall. You can perform a twist, but be mindful of *how* you are conceiving of the movement and what your various options are.

Double Spiral

It is now apparent that when performing what appears to be a simple Primary or Secondary action, in fact, all the spirals are involved in the support structure for the movement. Even while standing still, the body is suspended by the energetic double-spiral musculature if all aspects of the spiral are operating harmoniously. The spiral lens allows us to answer more sophisticated questions, to view movement and the body in a three-dimensional way, and to recognize that support and lengthening into movement are both involved in action and in stillness.

MOVEMENT EXPLORATION 5.9: DOUBLE SPIRAL STRAPS

Wrapping the body in straps provides a tactile reinforcement of the spirals' pathways, giving you a vivid sensation of the connections made throughout the body via the spiral musculature.

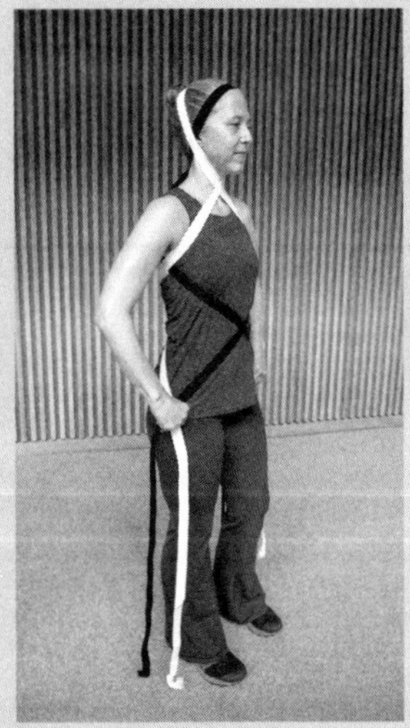

1. One strap from the back of head:

Hold a strap up and find the middle. Place the middle of the strap over the top of the head (but a little behind instead of directly in the middle). Place the strap over the ears, crisscrossing below the jaw/under the chin. Then pass the straps under the front of the armpits around to the back. They will join at the mid-back and crisscross again. From the mid-back, pass the straps around the sides of the body to end at the ASIS.

2. One strap from the front of head (upper forehead):

Hold a strap up and find the middle. Place the middle of the strap on the upper part of your forehead. Trace the two sides of the strap down over the ears to crisscross on the back of the neck. From the neck, pass under the armpits to cross in the front of the trunk just below the bottom of the sternum/solar plexus. Pass over the sides of the body and finish at the top of the back of the pelvis.

3. Mapping the spirals from head to pelvis and back, incorporating both previous explorations:

The next goal is to join explorations one and two so you can experience a whole double-spiral arrangement around the trunk. One easy way is to do each exploration with a different colored strap, holding the first strap in place while setting up the second, and then passing the ends of the straps through the groin/inner thigh area to tie them together at the sitz bones (ischial tuberosities).

Video: Double Spiral Straps

Another way to experience this is to use one long elastic strap to wrap the body in a loop in one long path that ends up reconnecting to itself.

MOVEMENT EXPLORATION 5.10:
MAPPING THE SPIRALS OF THE TRUNK

Before you start:

For an overview of the mapping, see the accompanying video at the end of the Movement Exploration.

You will need a partner and an elastic strap of at least four yards long.

Consider that in wrapping the person, you must keep a modicum of tension on the elastic throughout.

Step 1: Stand behind your partner. Place the strap on the back of their right shoulder and have them hold it with their left hand (across the front of their body). Guide the strap up on a diagonal to the left ear, over the front of the hairline, back down over the right ear, and down to crisscross the other strap at the back of the neck (C7).

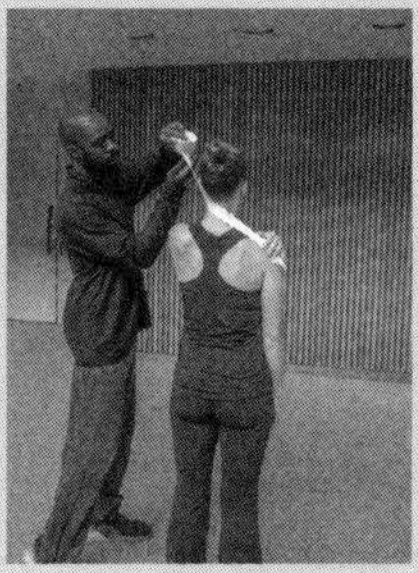

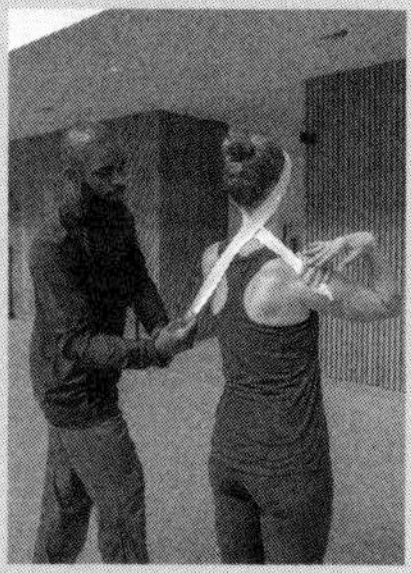

Step 2: Continue to stretch the strap from the base of the neck across the back, toward the left shoulder, passing under the arm, continuing around the side and diagonally down the front to end up at the front right hip (ASIS).

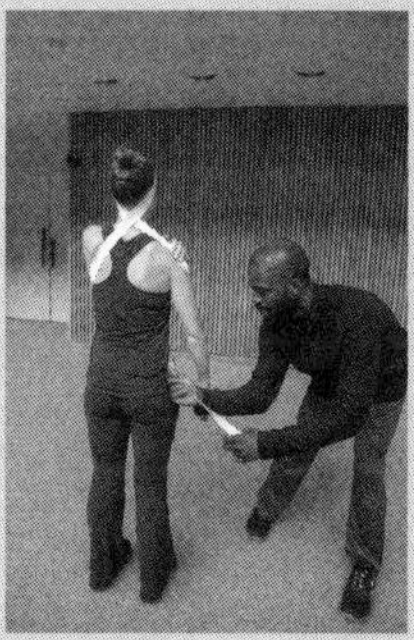

Step 3: From there, take the strap around the right hip toward the back, then between the legs, back up to the front, to cross over the band on the right hip (essentially forming a loop around the top of the right leg).

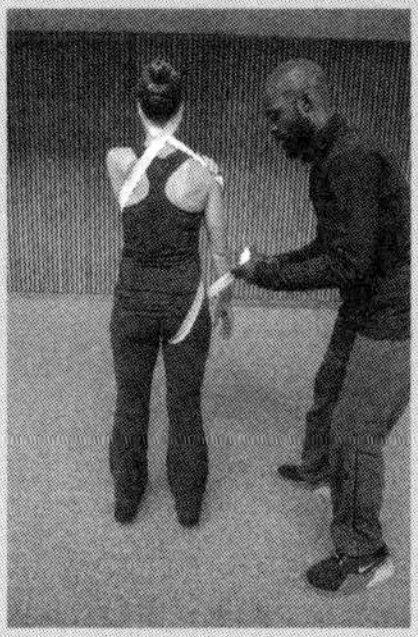

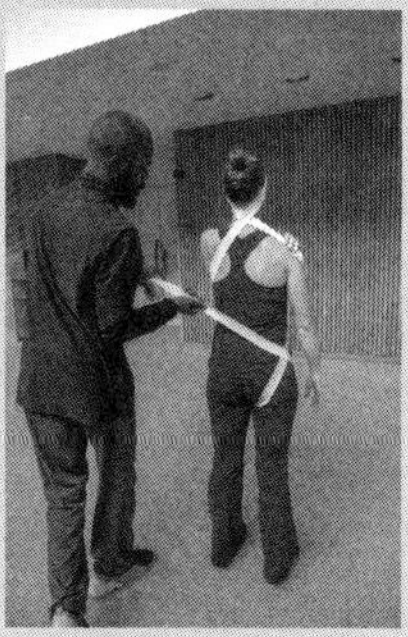

Step 4: Draw the strap diagonally up toward the inside of the left armpit, passing under the arm to the front of the body and then diagonally across the neck to the right ear.

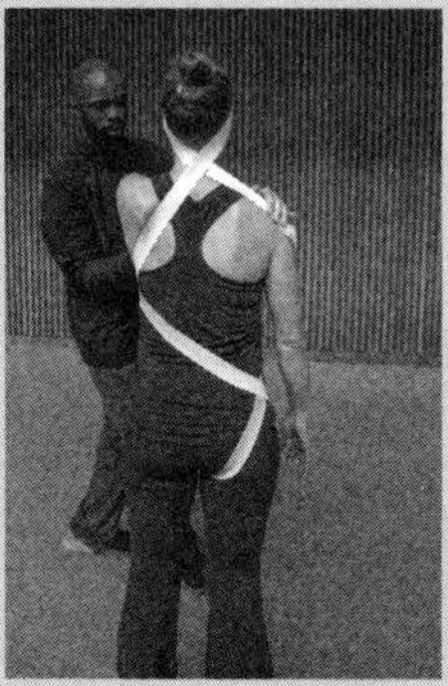

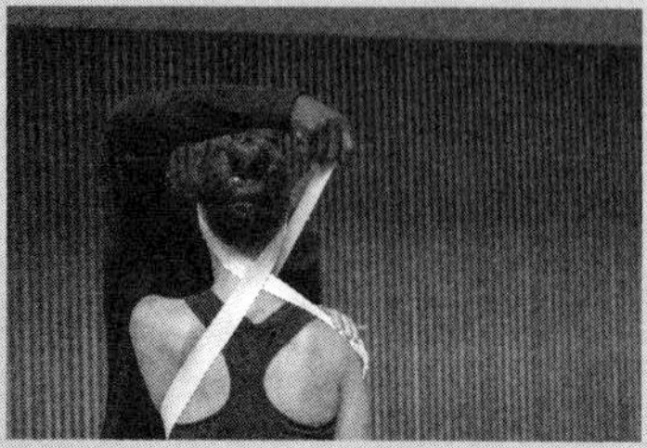

Step 5: Continue from the right ear over the back of the head to the left ear. Continue to the front of the neck and diagonally across the front of the body again, down to the right armpit.

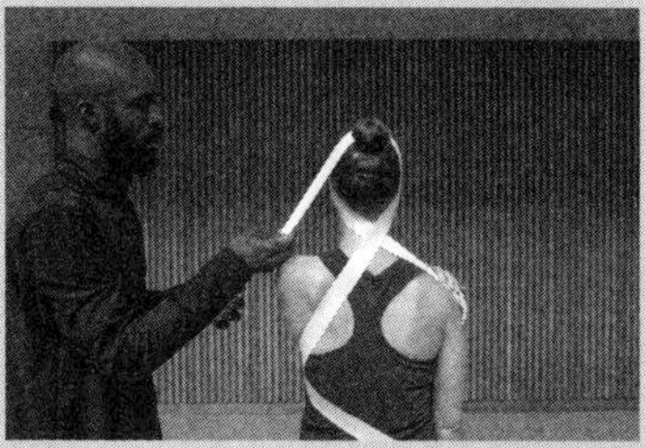

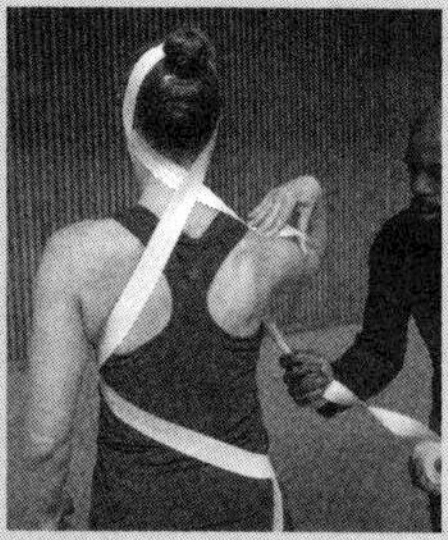

Step 6: Cross to the back under the right armpit, and diagonally across the back to the left hip.

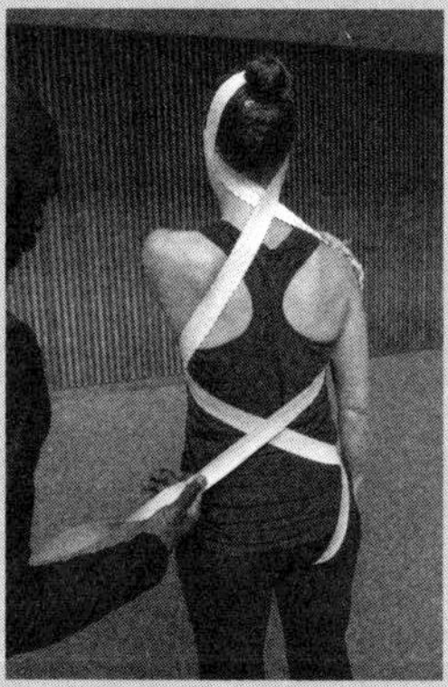

Step 7: "Loop" left leg by taking the strap from the left ASIS, passing it between the legs and back up around the bottom of the gluteals to come back up to the left hip.

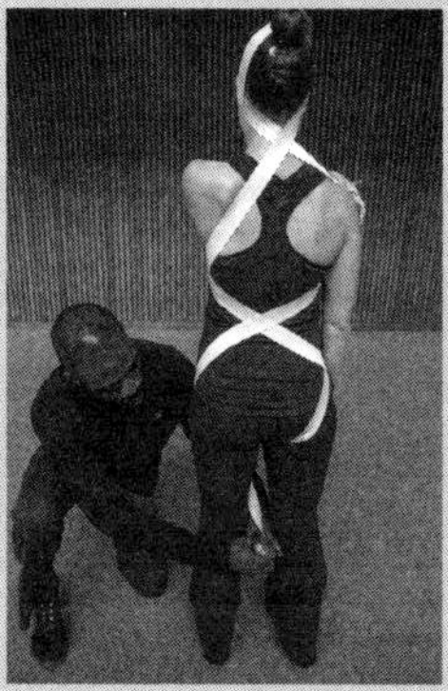

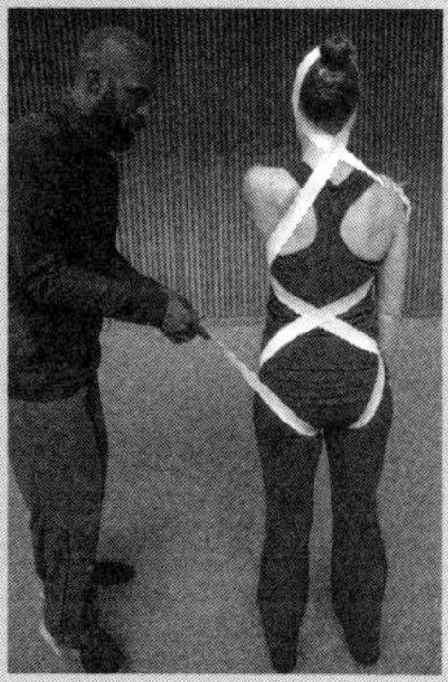

Step 8: From the left hip, once more, cross diagonally up the front of the trunk. Pass under the right arm and then connect the strap to the end your partner is holding (on the back). Ask your partner for the strap, and tie the two ends.

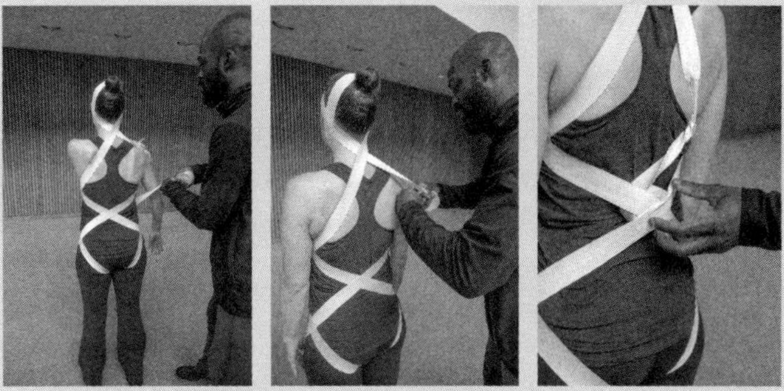

We now have a full three-dimensional double-spiral band encompassing the trunk.

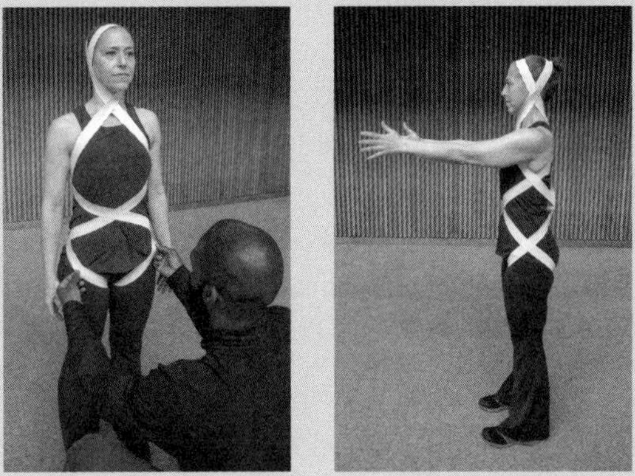

When wrapped in the double-spiral straps, try an activity of your choice: walk around your space, swing a golf club, cut a vegetable, play an instrument, pick up an object high and low, toss a ball, or dig up dirt.

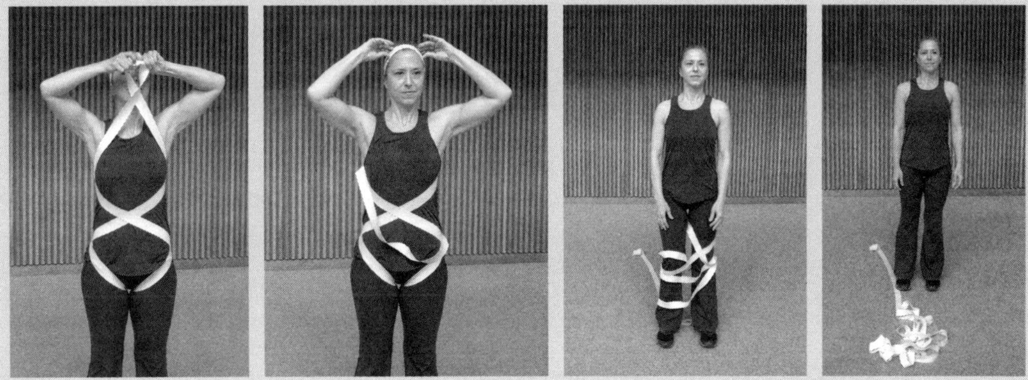

Getting out of the loop:

Take the strap at the back of the head and bring it forward to let it go. Take the strap from the front of the head to the back and let it go. While thinking "up," wiggle out of the elastics as they fall and then step carefully out of the loop. Once you take off the straps, are you more aware of the support of the spiral structure?

Video: Mapping the Spirals of the Trunk

Spirals in the Limbs

The muscular spiral arrangement continues through the limbs as well as the torso. In evolutionary thought, limbs are a development from fishes' lower gills, which transformed into fins and later limbs in land animals (Shubin 2008). From a Framework for Integration perspective, limbs are inexorably related to the trunk, Engaging and Resetting rhythmically as they weave through spiral patterns.

Arms

As we illustrated in Movement Exploration 4.1, the arms respond to Primary by rotating in, and they rotate out as you look up toward Secondary. We can also initiate this movement from the fingertips.

MOVEMENT EXPLORATION 5.11:
ARM ROTATIONS TO INITIATE TORSO MOVEMENT

From standing, raise the arms to the sides, and start to turn both arms inward, beginning from the fingers, and allowing the lower arm, then the upper arm to follow. Your torso will respond by curving forward into Primary. To enhance this experience, let the knees bend as well. Now initiating with the fingers, turn the arms outward, letting the movement sequence into the torso and head, so that you end up looking up toward the ceiling. As you do that, allow the knees to straighten.

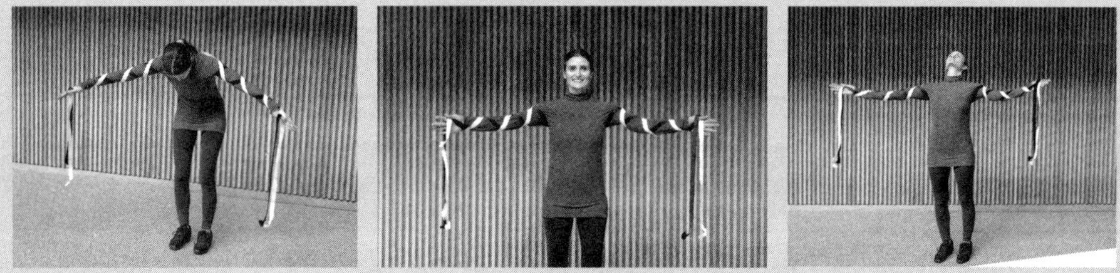

This movement can be initiated either way—from the head or the fingers—there is no correct way of doing it. In either case, you can experience the connectivity between the torso and the arms, as the double spiral comes into play.

MOVEMENT EXPLORATION 5.12: FISH ARMS WHILE STANDING

This movement sequence is a variation of "fish arms" from the Dart Procedures, and it further explores the arm rotations supported by the rest of the body.

Begin standing, with feet under your hip joints, and arms down by your sides. You will be raising the arms sideward and then upward to end overhead. While doing this, you will be rotating the arms in and out along the way, leading with the fingertips. As you rotate your arms in, leading with the thumbs, allow your gaze to go down slightly, and your weight to shift a little bit back on your feet. As you rotate your arms out, leading with your little fingers, allow the gaze to go up slightly, and your weight to shift a little bit forward on your feet. With each rotation the arms can continue to rise. Keep in mind, as you do this arm movement, that the arms' pathway should be slightly in front of the body, so that you can see your hands in your peripheral vision. Also, make sure you are not locking or straightening your elbows or knees.

Ultimately, the arms will end up overhead but slightly in front of your body, with the lower arms pronated, elbows bent, and the back of the wrists touching. You will be in a slight Primary. Notice how the corresponding movement of the body supports and provides more ease in the movement of the arms.

◎ Video: Fish Arms While Standing

The accompanying video "Straps on Arms Double Spirals" shows the integration of the Primary and Secondary spirals from arm to arm across the back, allowing us to see the arms' effect on the spine.

◎ Video: Straps on Arms Double Spirals

It is also possible to counterspiral the arms, so that the upper arm is outwardly rotating while the forearm is inwardly rotating, or vice versa.

MOVEMENT EXPLORATION 5.13:
DOUBLE SPIRALS OF ARMS—UPPER AGAINST LOWER, BOTH WAYS

Raise your right arm forward, approximately parallel to the floor. With your left hand, gently massage your upper arm in an outward direction, allowing the whole arm to follow that direction, starting from the top and working down to the elbow in three to four strokes. Repeat that a few times. Maintaining the outward direction of the upper arm, gently massage the lower arm in an inward direction so that the palm faces down, starting from the elbow and working down toward the wrist. Repeat a few times.

Once you have finished, repeat with the other arm.

◎ Video: Double Spirals of Arms—Upper Against Lower, Both Ways

Notice whether this feels different than before you gave yourself the directions.

Just as the body's double-spiral mechanism provides support for the torso, the counterspirals in the arms offer support without excessive effort, offering a way to distribute the workload throughout the upper torso. With this in mind, take a look at your everyday and specific activities that involve arms, noticing where this double spiral of the arms can be supportive.

Connectivity of Hand to the Opposite Hip

If you extend the design of the trunk's double spiral, as explained in Movement Exploration 5.10, into the arms, you can see that the movement of an arm would have a direct relationship to the opposite hip.

MOVEMENT EXPLORATION 5.14: HIP TO FINGERS SPIRAL PATHWAY

Using a yoga strap, tie one end around the top of your left thigh. Bring the strap across the back and diagonally up to your right armpit, passing it under and toward the front. Wrap the strap outwardly around the arm three times, going from the armpit to the wrist on the little finger side, and pass it into the palm to hold on to it.

Extend the arm in front of you to feel the tension across your back and all the way to your left hip. Outwardly rotate your arm and re-extend it, keeping the tension even across the whole strap. While the arm is extended, see if you can transfer the weight onto the right leg and pick up the left leg behind you.

Video: Hip to Fingers Spiral Pathway

Another movement to try is to punch the right arm, feeling the back and the hip participate. The weight shifts to the right foot as you punch and Resets as you release from the punch. If you try to stay on two legs, that might feel uncomfortable. For ballet dancers, this is very informative for performing an *arabesque* or *effacé*, clearly showing the spiral connection between the right fingers/hand and the left hip. This connectivity is at play in many activities, from playing the violin, to swinging a tennis racket, to simply reaching up for a plate or glass in your kitchen cupboard.

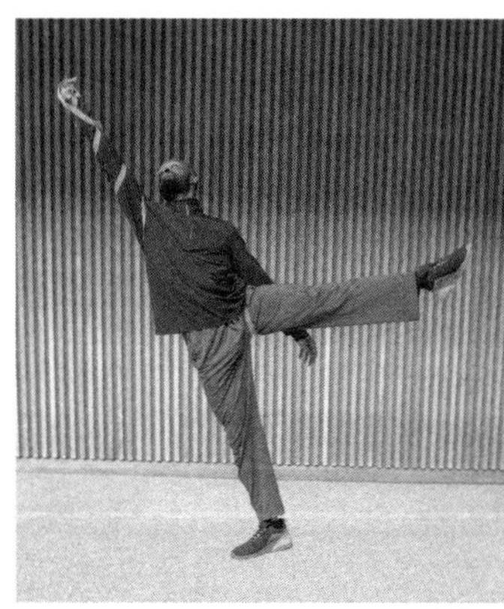

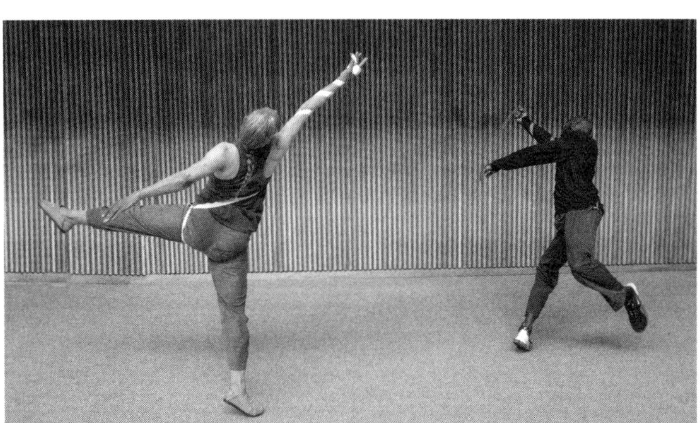

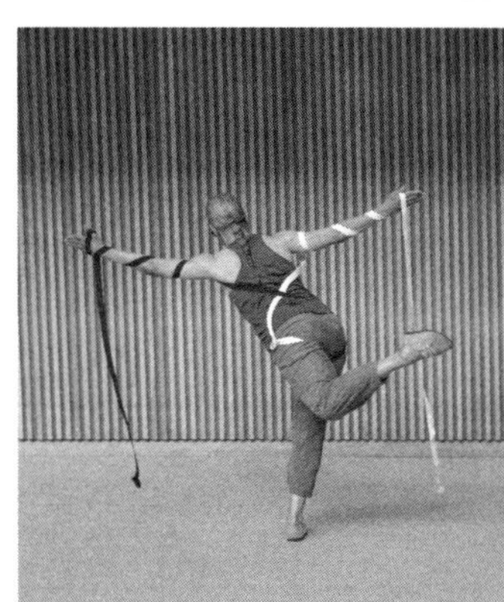

Legs

While writing *Dance and the Alexander Technique,* we hesitated to discuss the relationship we observed between the spiraling torso and the lower limbs, particularly the feet and ankles. Preconceived notions in dance and other movement practices often dictate an idea of maintaining symmetry in the ankles despite weight shifts, rotations, and locomotor activities. Dance training often advocates consistent lifting of the arches of the feet as a place of neutrality and support, or countering the tendency to pronate or collapse. It has become apparent to us that the effort to keep the feet and ankles locked into a "place" is detrimental in the long run.

As previously discussed, spiraling transfers our weight, and consequently, the legs respond and the feet either pronate or supinate. As we discovered in Movement Exploration 5.8, analogously, actions in the upper and lower leg lead to pronating and supinating patterns that can be experienced as lengthening or shortening, depending on the action. While they might not seem as supple as your arms, your legs have the capacity to be similarly responsive. This seems obvious until we confront strongly held beliefs about the stability we feel the legs must provide in standing, when in fact, support comes mainly from the torso in complex conversation with the legs. For a clearer illustration of this, go to the link for mapping trunk and leg spirals with bands (see video link below).

Video: Mapping of the Trunk and Legs

> As a former competitive gymnast turned gymnastics coach, learning how to land was emphasized, specifically because gymnasts generally land from great heights. Much like the way I was coached, when I taught young girls how to land, I allowed them to wobble and find their balance and stability in their own time; I emphasized the role that the ankles play in this. I said, "The wiggles and jiggles are the body's way of figuring out how not to fall. This will happen faster the more you practice!" When they landed in their chair position with arms stretched out in front, executing a "stick it," I would verbally cue the girls to let their ankles and toes be expansive—not gripped—and mobile to quickly adapt to the sudden stop in momentum and speed and the wiggles that came with them. After, I'd go up to them and ask them to close their eyes so I could check their balance—lightly pushing their pelvis around as they allowed and adjusted to the exterior mobility to find stability and, therefore, safe practices for landing from high up in the future.
>
> —Nik Owens, Dance graduate student, University of Illinois

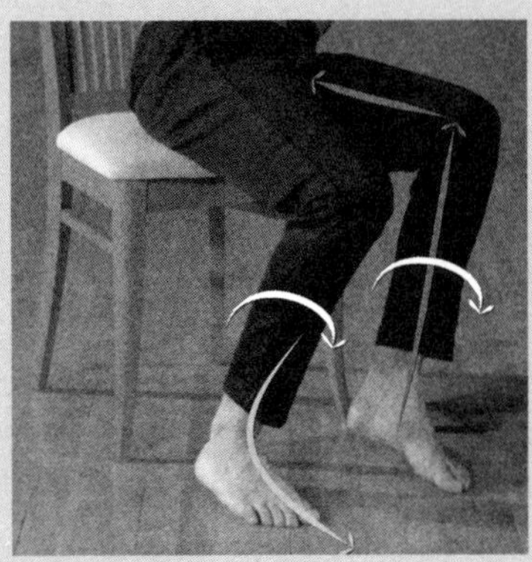

MOVEMENT EXPLORATION 5.15: SPIRALS TO EXPLORE FEET/ANKLES/KNEES/HIPS CONNECTION

Sit at the edge of your chair. Start by looking left, making sure your weight transfers onto your left hip as you keep spiraling until you are looking behind yourself. At the apex of the spiral, the left foot supinates and the right foot pronates (if not interfered with). Notice that the two legs are doing different activities. As the hip brings you back to balance on both sitz bones, the legs will sequentially return to the starting position. Repeat this on the other side and make note of differences.

MOVEMENT EXPLORATION 5.16: SPIRAL FROM SITTING WITH LEGS IN FRONT

Sit on the floor with your legs extended to the front. If this is difficult for you, you can raise your pelvis by sitting on a cushion or a block. Imagine someone is calling you from behind, and you want to turn your head to the right to look. As you do, allow your weight to transfer to your right hip and you can use your arms to help support you. Your right shoulder is opening in Secondary while your left shoulder is moving toward Primary, so it makes sense to bring your left arm forward. Turning your attention to the legs, the right leg will turn out, and the foot will supinate, while the left leg turns in and the left foot pronates. Be sure you are not locking your knees. Notice differences between the two legs—they have different responses to the spiral. The left leg is lengthening while the right leg is softening.

Video: Spiral from Sitting with Legs in Front

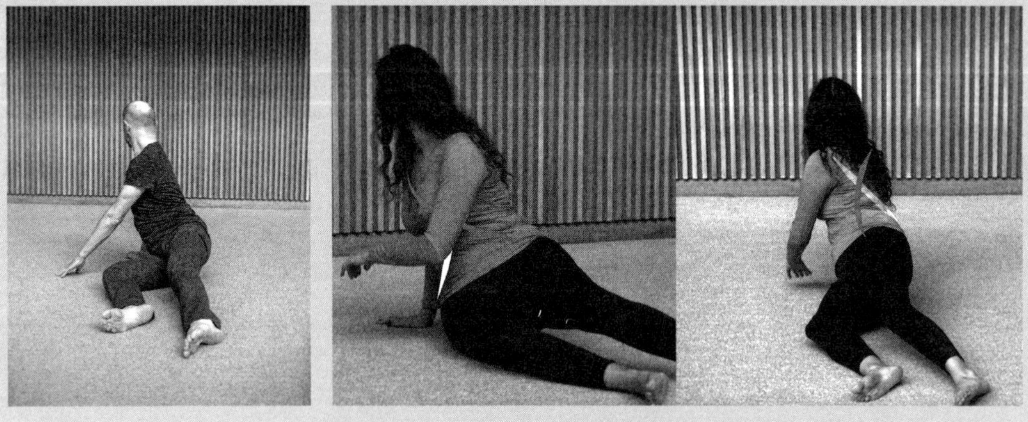

Just as the arms are responsive to the spirals in the trunk, so are the legs. Looking down encourages a gentle supination of the feet, while looking up stimulates a slight pronation. The feet and ankles should be responsive to the activities of the rest of the body rather than held rigidly. The ankles and feet are designed to help you navigate uneven terrain, adjust to weight shifting, and participate in propulsion in any direction.

Summary

The Complex Model—approaching the body and movement through a spiral lens—looks at our body in a more sophisticated way, more representative of our structure and movement capabilities. While the Simple Model provides building blocks for this more complicated, three-dimensional outlook, it doesn't reveal the whole picture. The spiral has the potential to generate movement, and the interweaving spirals provide support in a dynamic rather than static way.

Symmetry is usually considered desirable when it comes to looking at the body, and in fact, can become an obsession in terms of trying to even out the twists and asymmetries that exist in all of us. This viewpoint can lead to treating the trunk as a block—we try to square it off, thinking that holding it is the only way to control it. This pressure to be symmetrical interrupts the flow of interaction between the spirals.

Granted, we all have imbalances and may favor spiraling toward one side more than the other. These twists are often the result of habitual preferences, dominant handedness, or occupational movement patterns, such as a violinist who necessarily spends a great deal of time rotated toward one side. These types of habitual spirals affect the whole body, which then in turn reinforce the preferred twist. Attempts at fixing the parts bypasses the general idea that the system comprises two spirals in balance with each other. To work on one spiral and allow it to Reset, and then to work on the other spiral, allowing it to Reset, lets you see the small local interferences in the limbs—the arms, the feet, the legs—and then to Reset the broader interferences in the spine. Gradually you may find that you are able to undo some of these previously unrecognized holding patterns by working with the spirals.

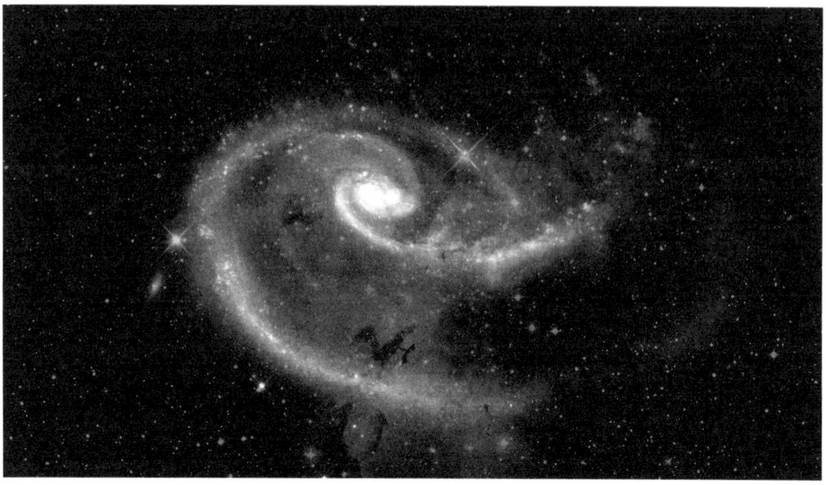

> **[In] examples ranging from the spiral nebulae to the human cochlea, and from the propagation of sound to the propulsion of solid bodies, . . . all things move spirally and all growth is helical.**
>
> **—Raymond Dart**

We encourage you to observe instances when using the spiral could enhance and/or clarify the movement you are doing. For example, how can the spiral assist you in turning your head to look both ways before you cross the street, or to back up the car? How can engaging in the full spiral increase your range of motion for a baseball or golf swing? How does the spiral work for shifting weight in something simple, like walking? Many examples are in Chapters Fourteen and Fifteen, but do take some time to explore this as you go about your daily activities and see what you discover as well.

Chapter 6

Timing Matters

This chapter highlights one of the most fundamental aspects of movement: timing. Timing, as pointed to in the accompanying quotes, encompasses speed, phrasing, deciding on *when* but also *how* we choose to perform any movement. Timing and movement quality are inextricably linked.

Timing: The selecting of the best time or speed for doing something in order to achieve the desired or maximum result.

—Dictionary.com

The choice, judgment, or control of when something should be done. "One of the secrets of golf is good timing."

—The Oxford English Dictionary

MOVEMENT EXPLORATION 6.1: PHRASING TYPES[1]

1. Even phrasing

Describe what you ate for breakfast this morning to someone, but do so with absolutely no inflection. Keep all the words at the same pitch and with no rhythmic variation.

Now try the same type of even phrasing in movement. Try moving with no emphasis or variation in timing. Keep it as even in flow as you can. Observe how this even flow made you feel, whether you enjoyed this activity, and what came to mind.

2. Impulsive phrasing

Pretend to throw a ball to someone who is far away from you. This type of movement requires a burst of energy, a quick beginning, with a follow-through that is slower. Now improvise with this type of impulsive movement. The accent is at the beginning, where tension is gathered and then released suddenly. What types of movements can you think of that fit this kind of phrasing?

3. Impactful phrasing

Now do the reverse, pretending to catch a ball that is thrown to you from a distance. Then explore this type of movement, where the accent is at the end of the phrase. Another example of this type of phrasing would be pounding your fist on a table—literally making an impact. What other types of movement examples can you think of?

4. Resilient phrasing

For this exploration, first pretend that you are bouncing a ball. Feel the even up and down of this movement, responding to gravity. Then pretend that you *are* a ball. Let yourself be bounced. Feel the response to gravity and the resilience that is created. Notice the timing that is involved to make this image come to life.

Now try another type of resilience phrasing: a swing. Begin to swing your arm like a pendulum, letting your body respond as you swing it. This type of resilience has a different rhythm than the bouncing ball, but is still responsive to gravity, this time with a quick drop and a slower suspension. The meter that naturally emerges from this movement is an underlying three, so that you spend one count on the drop and two counts getting to and hovering on the up phase of the movement. Notice the inevitable drop that comes after suspending at the top of the arc.

It is obvious from the first movement exercise that it is almost impossible to speak without putting emphasis on any of the words. Phrasing is a natural outcome of wanting to express something. The same thing applies to movement. Each of these phrasing types makes different demands on the body in motion, and each one can be appropriate or inappropriate, depending on the situation or movement that you are doing. For example, a dancer is asked to perform a set of thirty-two jumps. If she finds the right timing that facilitates a bounce, so that she can rebound from the landing of one jump to the propulsion of the next, it will minimize the effort required for the jumps. Likewise, trying to throw a ball with even timing instead of using impulsive timing would not project the ball into space. We will explore this concept of tapping into the optimal timing throughout this chapter.

Gravity is the force which pulls everything towards the *centre* of the earth. In order to move, this force must be overcome by energy, and so we see a rhythmic cycle of waxing and waning energies. In all natural forms of life, deviations and disturbance may occur, but the underlying rhythmic harmony continues from day to day and season to season.

—Winearls, *Modern Dance: The Jooss-Leeder Method*

Rhythm

Rhythm is life, from seasonal, lunar, and solar cycles to the circadian rhythms that govern our bodies—our heartbeat and our breath. Even our brains have rhythm. Neuroscientist Nathan Urban explains, "Every cell in the brain has its own beat. Groups of brain cells synchronize when they need to get something done" (NPR 2014). Rhythm encompasses more than just a beat; it includes accent, meter, tempo, fluctuation, and flow. There is movement inherent in rhythm.

MOVEMENT EXPLORATION 6.2: WRITING YOUR NAME

If you have a pen and paper, write your signature. Then write it again with your finger in the air. Then write it again in the air, only bigger. Try it smaller. Try it on a different plane, such as over your head or below you. Try it with another body part such as your elbow. Play with this idea of writing your signature in many different ways. Notice: Was there a particular rhythm that you used when writing your name?

There is a specific motor program in your brain for writing your name, a set of muscle commands that allow for movement without the need for feedback. The muscles fire in the same proportion and with the same relative timing, whether it is with the hand, a different body part, bigger or smaller, faster or slower. This consistent relative timing of the movement pattern is the movement's fundamental "deep structure." Rhythm is an invariant feature in your motor program for writing your name (Schmidt and Lee 2014, 114). Surface features such as speed, size, and limb used are easy to alter, but the deeper relative-timing structure is difficult to change.

Musicality

In the context of dance, we often talk about being musical when we dance. What does this mean? It is not about dancing on the beat or being accurate, but rather, making qualitative choices about phrasing and timing within a certain musical structure, so that the dancer artfully interacts with the music. In fact, a dancer does not need to dance to music to be musical. One can dance in silence but still conjure up a rhythm and melody within the movement. Melody has rising and falling pitches and intervals, giving flavor and texture to the rhythms inside it. These characteristics can apply to all types of movement, not just dance.

In *Musicophilia,* Oliver Sacks tells a story of being injured on a mountain, not able to get himself down. He eventually made his way down by thinking of a marching song with a strong heave on each beat. "Before this I had muscled myself along; now with the beat, I was musicked along. Without this synchronization of music and movement, the auditory with the motor, I could never have made my way down the mountain." After surgery, he forgot how to walk. He tried to consciously walk (step by step)—that didn't work very well. But when he thought of a piece of music, the natural rhythm and melody of walking came back to him, and "along with this, the feeling of my leg as alive, as part of me once again. I suddenly 'remembered' how to walk" (Sacks 2008, 234).

Humans have incredibly accurate memories for tempo and rhythm. Keeping time physically and mentally depends on interactions between the auditory and the dorsal premotor cortex, and it is only in the human brain that a functional connection between these two cortical areas exists. These sensory and motor activations are precisely integrated with each other (Sacks, 240). Sacks also states, "Listening to music or imagining it, even without any overt movement or keeping time, activates the motor cortex and subcortical motor systems. Thus, the imagination of music, of rhythm, may be as potent, neurally, as actually listening to it. Rhythm in this sense, the integration of sound and movement, can play a great role in coordinating and invigorating basic locomotor movement" (2008, 241).

Resilience

> In developing skill, one should learn to exploit the passive dynamics of the body—essentially, the energy and motion that come for free with the help of physics. The movement becomes maximally skilled in terms of effectiveness, and efficiency (minimum outlay of energy).
> —From Nicholai Bernstein's *Theory of Stages of Learning* (Schmidt and Lee 2014, 211)

This thought is echoed by Alexander Technique teacher and musician Pedro De Alcantara:

> Finding the proper rhythm for your actions means letting the rhythm itself do most of the work for you. Riding the rhythmic release of energy inherent in movement requires a lot less physical effort than "doing" and "controlling."
> —Pedro De Alcantara, *Integrated Practice: Coordination, Rhythm and Sound*

In an effort to control, we may purposely or unconsciously omit any momentum or swing in the movement. In other words, the movement is continual Engagement with no Reset. This might be appropriate for something like strength training, but it doesn't necessarily lend itself to everyday movement or skilled dance or athletic movements. Going back to the earlier movement exploration of different phrasing types, *even* movement phrasing does not necessarily equal *ease* of movement. It depends on the situation. Sometimes trying to even out the timing kills the quality of the spring that we are looking to uncover.

The word "spring" means "to rise, leap, move, or act suddenly and swiftly, as by a sudden dart or thrust forward or outward, or being suddenly released from a coiled or constrained position," or "a sudden movement caused by the release of something elastic" (Dictionary.com). Notice that these definitions emphasize the timing involved in the release of the coil.

MOVEMENT EXPLORATION 6.3:
THE RESILIENCE OF THE STRUCTURE

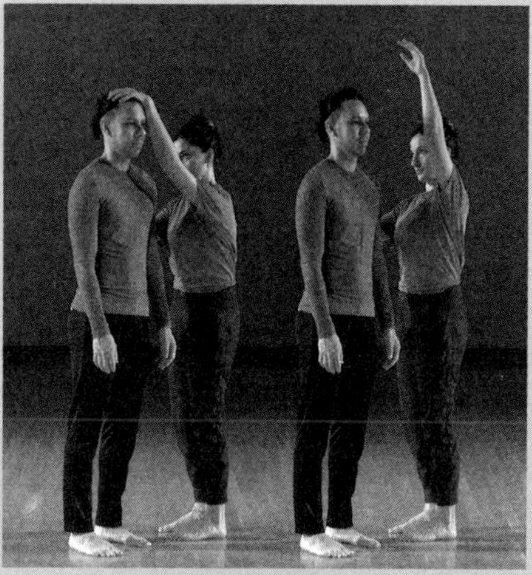

This movement exploration is designed to be done with a partner, but if no one is available, you can try it on yourself. Standing beside your partner, and facing them, put your front hand on the top of their head. (If you are working alone, put both hands on the top of your own head.) Make sure you place your hands right on top—neither too far forward nor too far back. The aim is to be able to exert pressure on the head straight through the spine into the feet. If your hands are too far back, you will encourage too much Secondary. If too far forward, you will encourage too much Primary. Try to find a balance. Then press down on the head with a degree of firmness, very slightly engaging Primary. The person whose head is being pressed down needs to resist the pressure. Then suddenly, release your hands. Hopefully you will see your partner bounce up, Resetting from the Engagement. It may be subtle, but if done correctly, it is usually quite apparent. Notice that you need to release with quickness. If you release slowly, you will not get the bounce.

Video: The Resilience of the Structure

Resilience is inherent in our system. Tapping into this resilience gives us the chance to, as Alexander said, "let the right thing do itself" (Carrington 1999).

MOVEMENT EXPLORATION 6.4: REVISIT THE BOUNCE

Practice the movement exploration from the beginning of this chapter: resilient phrasing, where you bounced a ball, an imaginary ball, and then yourself as a ball. This time, focus more on the timing involved. Feel how the interplay with gravity can assist you in rebounding from the floor.

In this movement exploration we become aware of our relationship with gravity, and how to access it to facilitate the action. Tapping into the rhythm of this movement is an example of movement efficiency.

Double Spiral as a Launchpad to Musicality

We explored spirals in Chapter Five. Here we revisit the spiral through the lens of rhythm.

MOVEMENT EXPLORATION 6.5: SPIRAL ROLL

Lie on your belly, and then look around to your right, like a baby looking to see her mother behind her. Allow your weight to shift toward your left hip as you spiral. Keep looking until you inevitably roll over onto your back. Did you notice the Reset involved in this activity?

Go back to your belly and try rolling to your back again, but this time, make the timing as even as possible. What does this do to the movement?

Video: Spiral Roll—Even and Organic Phrasing

You might have noticed that it's impossible to do a spiral roll in an even timing. For the even timing to occur, you have to hold the body in a piece—like a log roll—and the spiral diminishes considerably. There is a rhythm involved in the spiral roll. In this case, the Secondary reach with the head/face takes longer than the Reset. Once you have achieved the wind-up phase, you don't need to use much force to roll. There is an interdependence of rhythm and efficient movement. One feeds the other. In this way, you can use rhythm to diagnose whether you are holding on unnecessarily in a situation where using the spiral would be most efficient.

Likewise, rhythm is embedded in the two interwoven spiral sheets of musculature surrounding the body, providing an inherent buoyancy to our structures. Both spirals are active at the same time to create a dynamic, responsive support system.

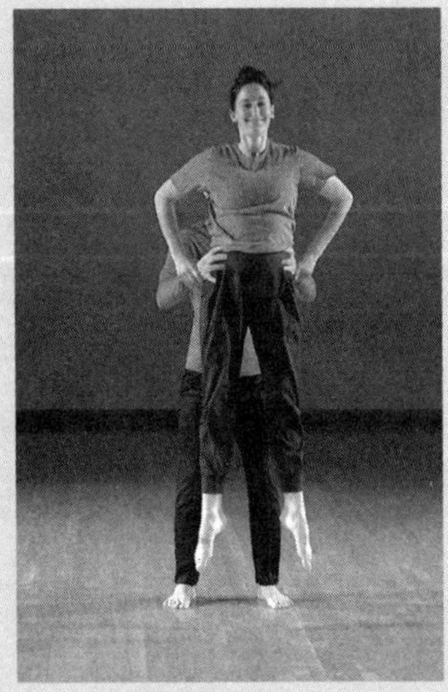

MOVEMENT EXPLORATION 6.6: BOUNCING TO JUMPING

Find a partner. Partner (A), stand with heels together and toes slightly turned out (first position). Partner (B), stand behind (A) in a wider position, and place your hands on either side of the top of (A)'s pelvis. (A), place your hands on top of (B)'s wrists.

For the next activity, (A), think of yourself as a solid structure, with the only movement available to you being the bending of the joints in your legs (hips, knees, ankles). You do not need to do anything to help in any way. You can think of yourself as a bouncy ball. (B), very gently start applying little pulses of pressure downward to make that ball (A) bounce. Continue bouncing (A) by pulsing downward, making the legs bend and release, until the heels start to lift off the floor in the release. No lifting from (B) is needed—just use the natural release from the push. (B), continue to increase the push, making larger bounces until (A) is leaving the floor. Make sure the push is gentle. It is just a small initiation that is repeated, not bigger and bigger initiations. Eventually (A) should be flying!

Video: Bouncing to Jumping

Notice that what is occurring here is the loading of Primary to allow the Secondary Reset to provide the lift off.

> The first time, I was trying to jump myself but I did not quite feel springiness when I thought, "I am going to jump giving more strength to go up" (like I do in a jump in ballet). My partner gave me the idea of releasing and just bending, feeling more bouncing instead of pushing up hard. And Becky also mentioned, "You do not need to do anything to help in any way." Yes, it was true! Thinking in this way also made me eventually fly! I was imagining I was a "flubber ball," or like a basketball with its rebounding. Letting my pelvis and legs bounce themselves made me more natural and elastic too! I felt some kind of different rhythmical balance as well. Very interesting! Super fun activity! After class, my friend asked me to try this again. At first I gave too much strength to fly: how dare me! Immediately, he said, "No, just pulse and bounce." I tried again, and I flew again! Yay!
>
> —Sojung Lim, Dance graduate student, University of Illinois

If you had to count this jump, would you choose an underlying duple (twos) or triple (threes) for this? Twos would refer to about the same amount of time spent down as up. So you would count it "one and two and." If you spent more time in the air than on the ground, you might count it "one and uh two and uh."

Irmgard Bartenieff claimed that in newborn babies, sucking produces a wave-like rhythm, and biting an angular rhythm (Bartenieff 1982, 71). Alex Murray claims that when the baby nurses, it sucks rhythmically if it's a happy baby. If he sucks once and breathes in/out, it's a rhythm of two. If he breathes in between every two sucks, it's a rhythm of three. Twos and threes are built into our systems right from the beginning. In movement, twos and threes are differentiated by the back-and-forth nature of twos, like a march, and the circularity of the threes, like a waltz or a swing.

MOVEMENT EXPLORATION 6.7: WALKING IN TWOS AND THREES

Try walking in an even meter, like a march. If you have space, do this for a period of time to really get into the rhythm of it. Then try another version of a walk that is in a three.

Video: Walking in Twos and Threes

What differences do you notice? Which did you prefer? One is not better than the other, but one might be more useful in certain situations. Did focusing on the rhythm make the walking seem easier? Did you find times when you could Engage more and then Reset from that Engagement? Did you notice the spirals as you walked?

Upbeat

In the previous walking exercise, did you notice the movement in between the steps? The moment you take the weight on the foot, or the landing phase, we might call the downbeat. The movement in between might be considered an upbeat. Upbeat can refer to a preparation for a movement, or an unaccented beat that immediately precedes a downbeat. We also use the term to describe someone who is optimistic or cheerful. Bartenieff discusses upbeat as a "preparatory movement that sometimes consists of effort elements that are opposite of those in the main statement" (Bartenieff 1982, 71). For example, a light upbeat for a strong statement. Or you might think of the opposite spatial direction. "In preparing a horse for a jump, the rider starts the pre-jump with a slight body and/or spatial retreating. That provides the rhythmic upbeat for the forward run and jump" (Bartenieff 1982, 73).

A conductor uses the upbeat to convey to the orchestra all the essential information for what is to follow. Leonard Bernstein argued that the conductor should be "reeling in the orchestra rather than acting as a metronome." The way to do this, he said, is to "obviously indicate what he wants before it is played" (Roberts 2017). Rhythmically, this upbeat moment can be extremely useful. It can give you a moment to think of what you are about to do and give thought to how the spiral is being used. This can help you to find the support and resilience needed for the movement. Knees bending before a jump provides an upbeat, even though the movement is in a downward direction. Often the upbeat is a breath, either an inhale or exhale, depending on the situation.

MOVEMENT EXPLORATION 6.8: SITTING AND STANDING

From a seated position, consider how you might stand up by, first, using a preparation where you allow yourself to sway a tiny bit backward in a rhythmic upbeat before standing. Here you are using a tiny bit of momentum to facilitate the movement.

Once you are standing, explore the idea of slightly tossing the head forward and up, and swaying forward over the toes a tiny bit, before bending at the hips to sit in the chair. After the initial head toss forward, you counterbalance the hips going backward with the head continuing to go forward. Once your hips land on the chair, you can bring the head over the pelvis to sit upright.

Video: Sitting and Standing

Reminding ourselves of an upbeat allows us to go up before moving, to decompress and elicit space inside the joints. It might seem counterintuitive, but a slight thought of "up" before bending the knees is useful in this way. The upbeat can also remind you to allow the neck to be free and to consider whether looking where you want to go can be helpful as a precursor to the movement. Considering the timing improves the function.

Interferences

> **An unrhythmic movement is lacking in economy of effort and so induces fatigue and strain.**
>
> **—Winearls, *Modern Dance: The Jooss-Leeder Method***

Although this quote is written in the context of modern dance, this concept can be applied to all types of activities. When, how, and why do we sometimes interfere with the rhythmic quality that would support the movements that we wish to do more easily and gracefully? The first step is recognizing some of the habits that may occur as we go about our daily activities. One particularly pernicious habit that many folks have is to hold their breath, especially when performing something difficult. Thinking about the rhythmic aspect of breathing may allow you to redirect this tendency to hold (see Chapter Eleven for a more thorough discussion of breathing).

Another instance where recognizing the rhythm of an activity is useful is in memorizing a movement pattern or sequence. Rather than thinking of each movement within the sequence as a separate entity, can you tie them together with rhythm?

MOVEMENT EXPLORATION 6.9: TEACHING FROM RHYTHM

Think of a daily activity, such as tying your shoe laces or a sequence of movements in a game or a sport, and then try teaching this sequence to someone else, just by showing them each movement in an isolated way, one after another. Then, develop a rhythm for this set of movements so that it becomes a "phrase." Teach it to someone by "singing" the rhythm of it first, and again as you go about showing it.

Most likely, the second way of teaching the movement sequence would be more successful for the learner.

If you are teaching a movement sequence or a task that involves movement, whether it is a dance class, a sports activity, an Alexander private lesson, or a repetitive task such as swimming, telegraphing the rhythm beforehand can be especially helpful in communicating the essence of the task. Also keep in mind that rhythm is an invariant feature of a motor program, so teaching something in the rhythm intended for the movement phrase is a key aspect of the movement itself.

Summary

Rhythmic logic promotes efficiency. Timing can play a key role in minimizing overuse of muscular force, or maintaining the tone required to move with power. If you are having problems with a particular movement or movement sequence, consider how you are performing it rhythmically. See if by changing the rhythm, you can find an easier way of doing it. Timing matters—both in designing and executing movement!

NOTE

1. The genesis of this phrasing material comes from Rudolf Laban's work, specifically as delineated in Vera Maletic's Ohio State University course workbook, *Dance Dynamics: Effort and Phrasing*, 2005.

Part Three

Framework for Integration, Integrated Model

Introduction

This part of the book delves into the Integrated Model, the unification of all the layers in Framework for Integration. In previous chapters, we discussed the importance of corresponding intents and actions in movement, as well as understanding the many possible interferences that can be observed through increased awareness of habits. Working with the Integrated Model depends first on clearly understanding the underlying Simple and Complex Models. As in any type of learning process, as you explore the Integrated Model, we encourage cycling back to the other models to keep remembering how they inform one another. While the Integrated Model is indeed more complex, there is no hierarchy of importance in the Framework. Now that we have explored rhythm's role in all bodily coordination, that awareness can also be factored into the increasing complexity.

Integration of Posture and Response: A Developmental Approach

Over years as we have taught this system in varied contexts, we have observed how students initially understand the Simple and Complex Models—particularly ideas of Primary and Secondary—through a shape-based lens or, more specifically, as the *shape* of posture. Given the cultural predominance of this lens in biomechanics, ergonomics, and aesthetic practices like dance, we understand the pull of this perspective and as a developmental stage, would never discourage or contradict it. But as we make our way into the Integrated Model, we reiterate that though Primary and Secondary can reflect certain shapes the body takes in snapshots of time, we are not working with posture as a "place" or notions of clear, static shapes, and as stated in Chapter Two, we maintain a resistance to the term "neutral" as an identifiable posture. Rather, we continue to point to how intention predicates and motivates the spectrum of movement (Primary and Secondary), see movement as an interplay of ever-shifting antagonistic action (spirals), and honor the built-in recuperative transitions we can notice and allow (Resets).

As defined by Merriam-Webster, we recognize that *posture,* as "the position or bearing of the body whether characteristic or assumed for a special purpose," can only serve as a guide. Having an awareness of posture by itself cannot help us know whether our response is appropriately calibrated to coping with varied mental/physical situations. We propose that if "good posture" is something to strive for, it is an ongoing, adaptive *process* that requires adjusting moment to moment. There are endless possibilities of "good posture" for any activity, and they are *outcomes* of that adaptive process. Any attempts to interfere with ongoing bodily (algo)rhythmic relationships is bound to limit our capacity to appropriately respond to stimuli. While a rudimentary understanding of posture as a static state might be helpful to a beginner, the Framework supports an evolving, self-teaching, adaptive rhythmic structure that supersedes shape. So far, we have introduced: the Simple and Complex Models, a growing vocabulary that includes the lexicon of Engagements and Resets and Primary and Secondary intents, and how all come together in spiraling arrangements. We hope these are now clear concepts. The Integrated Model brings it all together in a polyrhythmic symphony.

The Ball Is a Wheelchair: Evolution to the Integrated Model

In the fall of 2011, educators in the Peck School of the Arts at the University of Wisconsin-Milwaukee and contacts from Milwaukee Veterans' Affairs put together a lunch meeting so arts researchers could meet with physicians and other caregivers. As luck would have it, Luc was seated next to Jacklyn Justus, MSN, the spinal specialist in charge of the Zablocki Veterans' Administration Medical Center Spinal Cord Injury/Disorder Center, where veteran wheelchair athletes were treated. Their initial discussion evolved into two years of research that completely refined and redefined their understanding of how the athletes might be able to gain more access to their pelvises, as well as adapt to their limitations, in both daily and specialized athletic movements.

Their first conversations highlighted the difficulties contemporary veterans found themselves facing with an overall increased time in the wheelchair. Over the twentieth and twenty-first centuries, spinal injury and paralysis medical interventions have become more sophisticated, increasing quality of life and longevity. A longer life in a wheelchair means that veterans and others now face more issues resulting from using the chair itself. These challenges were further amplified for veteran athletes working at the edges of their balance and range of motion. The discussions with Jacklyn and working with the athletes sparked Luc's continuing interest in the relationship of development to design. He and Jacklyn came to the agreement that three areas of wheelchair design could use improvement: the wheels, the seat, and the mechanisms by which the athletes could become aware of their pelvises during activities, even if they had little to no sensation. During those years, Jacklyn and Luc were able to explore and work on two of those goals.

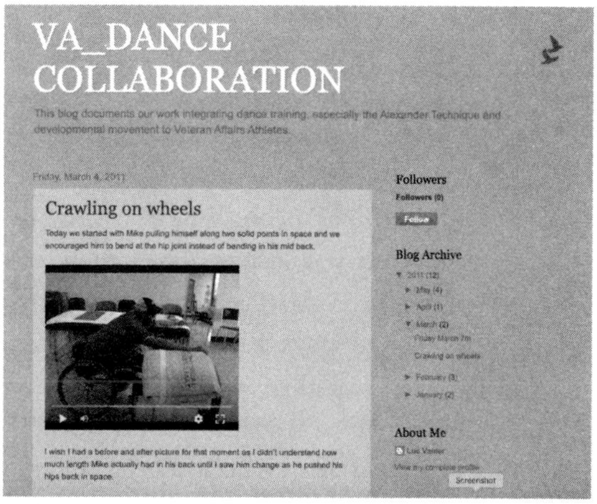

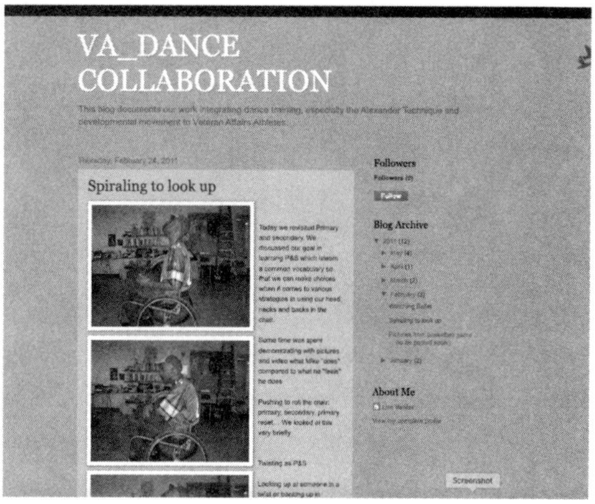

Screen captures of Luc's blog archiving his work with veteran and wheelchair athlete Michael Thomas. Mike's "crawling" and spiraling in his chair translated to the Framework for Integration's work on the physioballs.

The Wheels

After taking some time to experience the feeling of being in a wheelchair, Luc saw that *pushing* the wheels to go forward in space was actually counter to developmental patterns of forward locomotion. Growing babies learn to *pull* with their arms and upper bodies to go forward in space (as the lower body pushes), first on their bellies and then all fours (see Chapter Four). Also, pulling with the front legs is a common way for quadrupedal animals to move forward in space and yet, anyone in a wheelchair is automatically asked to push the wheels to move forward. In early developmental movement, pushing from the arms and upper body normally sends the baby backward in space. Seeing this developmental coordination incongruence, Luc noticed that pushing while looking up to see where one is going could negatively impact the neck and arms, especially the shoulder cuff area. He and Jacklyn agreed that reverse wheels might be beneficial; they soon became available.

The Seat

A wheelchair is a personal piece of equipment specifically fitted to its user. Unsurprisingly, the design is affected, in part, by the desire to keep its seated occupant safe. When in long-term use by active movers, unfortunately, "safety" features that are included for legal/liability reasons can restrict the freedom available for those using the chairs, while also forcing unhelpful or damaging movement habits. Luc's work and explorations with one veteran, an extraordinary individual named Mike, yielded the idea that an adaptable, moving seat could help reduce overwork in the upper part of the spine by providing counterbalance at the base of the spine/pelvis, where people with paralysis are not capable of feeling their hip joints or lower backs.

Another relevant observation was that for most users, the wheels of the wheelchair become de facto hip joints. However, most cannot fully access their substitute "hips" because the wheelchair design banks them far back in the chair, in a constant overall Primary orientation (trunk flexion) when they also need ample access to Secondary action (trunk extension and hyperextension for that pulling action). Having the most access to trunk orientation and action becomes even more important when an athlete in a wheelchair reaches sideways to, say, pick up a ball. Without the seat adapting to the activity or allowing the pelvis to move inside the stability of the chair, instead, the mover's spine adapts where the hip joints would normally shift. This over-substitution of spine for pelvis can create serious issues over years. In response to Luc and Jacklyn's observations, they created a seat that would move in response to activity. The seat would "escape" backward when the athlete reached forward, forward if the athlete looked up, and to the opposite side if they reached over the side. The design was rudimentary but an improvement to the ordinarily fixed state of the seat.

Sensory Help

The last part of the project and developing the theory ultimately changed how we approached teaching dancers and Alexander Technique teachers. In brief: We agreed that if someone could not feel a weight transfer from one side of the pelvis to the other, over time, it would negatively affect their body and use of the chair. Luc worked with researchers at the University of Wisconsin-Milwaukee to develop a weight-sensing system that would be integrated into the chair's seat, with haptic vibration devices that could be felt by the upper body, thus allowing wheelchair users to know whether their weight was transferring from one wheel to the other. Knowing this would help a user extend their spine as much as they could, and maybe strengthen and expand whatever unused capacity they had. Due to various deterrents, they were not able to finish this design. However, the design revealed that regardless of ability, understanding how weight is transferred from hip to hip took on new importance. One hip works (Engages) while the other rests (Resets), and the vital relationship between head and pelvis becomes even more apparent.

What Was Learned

It is important to note that working with people who have differently abled access to their bodies who accomplish their movement dreams and goals is inspiring. Over the years we learned so much from our work with Mike and others about successful strategies to avoid amplifying habits that can add extra struggle or difficulty in a wheelchair. Our lessons were documented and tested in our budding Framework for Integration. We extend a deep sense of gratitude to these incredible people for allowing us to work with them and learn from their strength and inventiveness. Thanks to these interactions, in our consequent teaching, we started to work with physioballs to illustrate people's tendencies to overuse parts of their spines rather than understanding the dynamic relationship between the pelvis and the head. These explorations created the third model in the Framework, the Integrated Model, and have grown and evolved ever since.

Physioballs

In the previous chapters you have seen how elastic and cloth straps (which started as masking tape and scarves years ago) are now indispensable for illustrating our spiral musculature. After working with wheelchair athletes and dancers, we also added large physioballs. It became clear that the wheelchair itself was the most important feedback "prop" providing the movers ongoing insight about what was happening with the whole self. So we began using the physioballs as a substitute wheelchair "driven" by the pelvis—not as something to stabilize against (as is done in many conditioning and strength practices), but rather as a mobile tool that illustrates the dynamic actions and directions of the head, spine, and pelvis.

Props add important tactile feedback that helps the body/nervous system navigate varied relationships to space. As Alexander teachers, of particular interest to us is balancing perception between internal sensing (egocentric) and "object centered coordinates that are independent of oneself" (exocentric) (Pacini and Barnard 2021, 1). Chairs, physioballs, and straps add an important information loop that challenges movers' habitual responses to their environment and reorients them in real time to moment-by-moment needs, expanding access to options for new experiences, choices, and change.

In Part Three, we will explore varying activities on the physioballs, designed to deepen awareness and coordination of the head-to-pelvis relationship. On the ball, our work will go from simple to spiral, and then distinguish what we call Upper and Lower Triangles, always bringing back an attention to Engagements and Resets.

For this work, having a physioball available is optimal. Most athletic, "big box," and chain retailers have them at fairly affordable prices, and the ball often comes with an easy manual pump. We generally work on these size physioballs:

- 55cm—this is a good size for shorter individuals
- 65cm—if you have to choose one, this is a good generally medium size
- 75cm—this is a better size for taller individuals

The ball should be large enough to comfortably sit on without your hips being overly flexed or extended (close to a 90-degree angle). We work with physioballs that are slightly underinflated so the ball doesn't "push back" but rather receives your weight while also being firm enough to stay steadily balanced. We also recommend that you have a nonslip mat or surface under your feet (a yoga mat works great). For extra stability, you can add chairs or side tables on either side to help stabilize.

Alternatives:

- Sitting on a foam roller or a smaller 9 inch/25cm inflatable ball (such as a Pilates core ball) placed on the seat of a chair—though the range of motion will be much smaller and the foam roller will not allow for side-to-side activity as the ball does.
- If you have neither a ball nor a foam roller, sit in a chair, feet planted on the floor, and sense how you roll over your sitting bones or shift sideways from hip to hip as your orientation in the chair changes.

Since we spend so much time sitting every day, we sometimes lose a sense of how much the pelvis can still move. We hope the following work can enliven your understanding of how you can sit anywhere—in a chair, on a couch, on the floor, on a ball—and provide dynamic choices that encourage movement and freedom.

Chapter 7

Ball Work: Four Phases

> **I have never had a teacher tell me it is okay to move my pelvis to help me complete the exercise in a healthy way for my body. When we first started looking at this idea and using the exercise balls, I remember thinking, "This is so easy, I must be doing it right." But once I was led through explorations on the ball, I learned that the way I had been moving my body was creating a battle instead of having my whole body work together.**
>
> **—Katie Kovar, Dance undergraduate student, University of Florida**

As we start exploring work on the ball in the Integrated Model, it is important to remember that we have previously established that the head is connected to the pelvis through a complex mesh of double-spiral musculature. The Integrated Model is designed to help us consider that relationship in more depth. This model addresses the dynamic, antagonistic exchanges of the hip-to-head relationship while further delineating Resetting from Engagements in both Primary and Secondary activities, giving a more complete picture of the interplay between them.

The Ball

MOVEMENT EXPLORATION 7.1: GETTING USED TO THE BALL

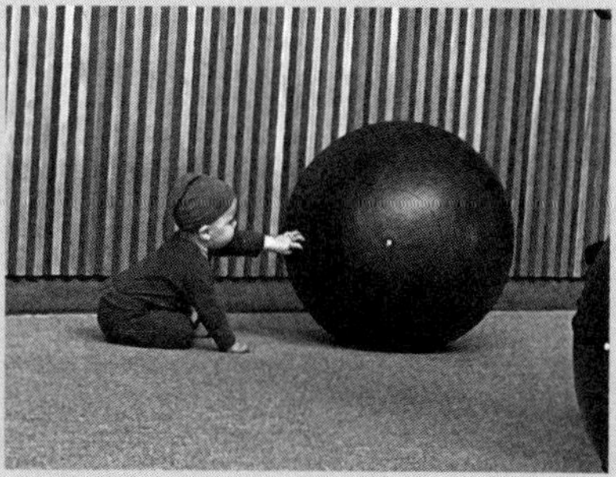

This movement exploration takes place on a physioball (refer to Part Three Introduction). It becomes easy to see the movement of the pelvis through the motion of the ball, as well as the inability to move the ball effectively. As suggested in the Introduction, we recommend a ball that is slightly underinflated and a nonslip mat or surface under your feet. Remember that raised surfaces on either side of you can help you balance and feel what is going

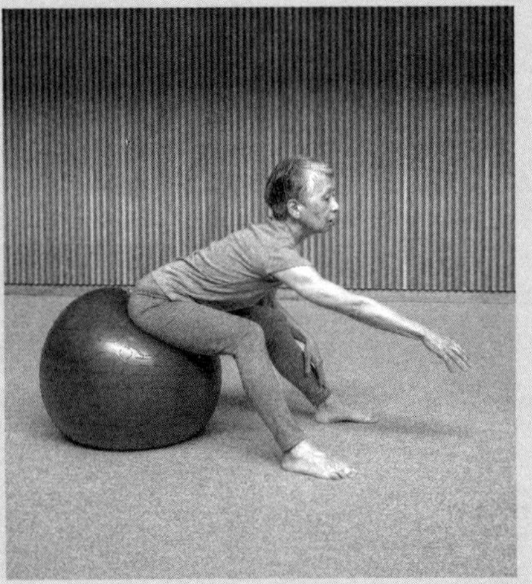

on with the ball. Our suggested alternatives (foam roller, small ball, or sensing sitz bones in the chair) may work with parts of this exploration, yielding more subtle sensation and feedback.

As you sit on the ball, aiming to stay upright, begin to play with moving your whole self in one piece (head to pelvis) forward and back on the ball. One direction might be easier than the other, and notice if your head or pelvis wants to get ahead of the other at any time in the movement. Once you feel coordinated and connected keeping them together, it's time to explore moving the head and the pelvis in opposition.

First, look down and touch the floor in front of you. Did the ball move and if so, where? Do this again and purposefully send the ball back into space as you touch the floor (the opposite direction your hands are reaching). Next, touch the floor to your right. Again, did the ball move and where? Do it again and allow the ball to "escape" to your left as you touch the floor on the right (again, ball in opposite direction). Did you try to keep your weight equally on both hips? Try it again but this time, make sure to shift your weight more to your right hip as you touch the floor on the right. Do the same to the left. Last, reach up as if to touch something above your head—you have probably guessed that the only direction we haven't sent the ball yet is forward. Reach up again, purposefully sending the ball forward. Note: In all directions, it helps to look in the direction where you are reaching.

Video: Getting Used to the Ball

This movement exercise is our dress rehearsal for the more complex movement ahead. We are now ready to apply the foundational concepts of Primary and Secondary. Later, in the upcoming explorations, we will layer in the concepts of Engagement and Reset.

The Four Phases

In the Alexander Technique, when we decide to stop or *inhibit* the habitual, we then redirect our energy and intention to freeing the spine in activity. The shorthand for this thought direction is usually known as "thinking up." Working with Primary and Secondary intents, coupled with our understanding of the spirals, we believe that "thinking up" is not limited by shape or direct relationship to gravity.

Having explored how movement of the ball is possible, we now delineate four specific, initial "phases" (or "ups") on the ball in either Primary or Secondary, with the ball going either forward or backward. Here, we are also adding a simple, fun shorthand we developed while teaching at Escola da Técnica Alexander do Rio de Janeiro (EsTAR) in Brazil. Every day, we could look out the studio window and, through a narrow corridor of other buildings, see the tempting view of the ocean. The imagery below is our homage to the beautiful landscape and people with whom we worked. Later, we'll demonstrate how these phases can be linked or affined to various activities.

Phase 1: Sitting on the ball in Primary, sending the ball forward
(Shorthand: *Resting in the beach chair*)

Phase 2: Looking down on the floor in Primary, sending the ball backward
(Shorthand: *Looking for your sandals*)

Phase 3: Looking out toward the horizon in Secondary, continuing to send the ball backward
(Shorthand: *Looking at the ocean*)

Phase 4: Looking up to the sky in Secondary, sending the ball forward
(Shorthand: *Looking for seagulls*)

As an awareness exercise, these Four Phases can now be linked to each other, one after another. We can begin noticing if we prefer one—or more—phases over others.

Video: The Four Linked Phases

In each of these Four Phases, there is the fundamental assertion that the pelvis is dynamically connected to the head through the double-spiral musculature. If you remember, spirals transfer weight, and in the double-spiral arrangement, double spirals working in coordination with each other will transfer weight forward or backward. Any time the head moves, the pelvis adjusts unless we interfere by immobilizing, anticipating, or misdirecting. Through the ball work, in various Engagements and Resets, the Integrated Model describes the crucial activity of the pelvis in relation to the head.

MOVEMENT EXPLORATION 7.2:
EXPLORING FOUR PHASES ON THE BALL

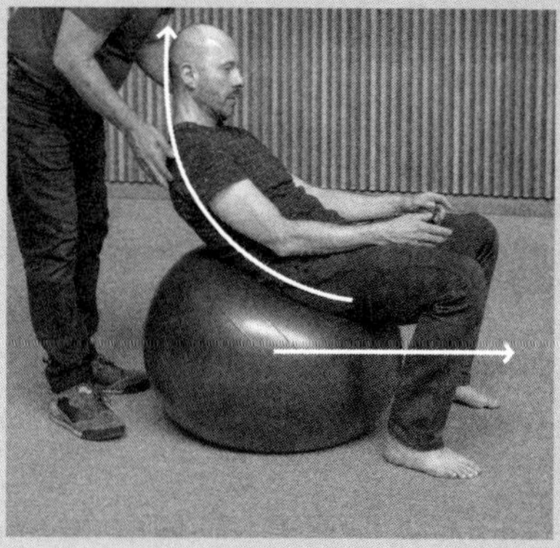

As you sit on the ball, explore these Four Phases of activity as described below. Remember that you can sit on the ball with support on either side so your arms can help you stabilize.

1. Primary Ball Forward or *resting in the beach chair*: Sit on the ball, allowing it to roll forward slightly as your torso stays back (as if you are relaxing back in that beach chair). Your hips will be forward of your head. Release any arch you may feel in your lower back, soften the front of the body (toward "hollowing"), allow the front of your ankles to soften (dorsiflex), and let your knees bend and direct more forward in space. Depending on the size of the ball and your height, your torso may feel quite far back in space.

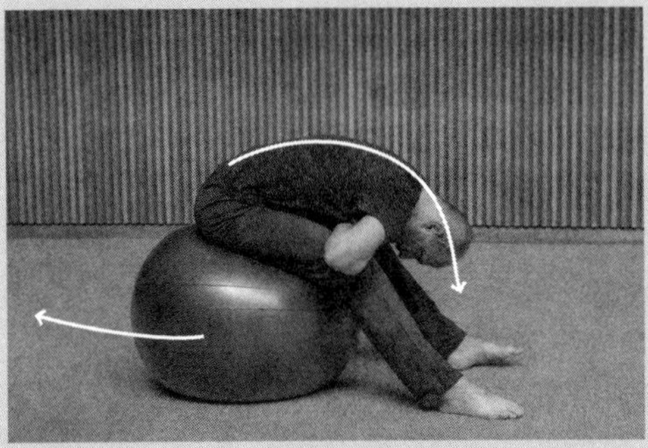

2. Primary Ball Back or *looking for your sandals*: If you look down toward your sternum and curl forward, we expect the ball to move backward. This demonstrates in a coordinated manner that the hips go back while the head goes forward. The hips respond to the intention and movement of the head and allow for a balance between them. Notice the difference between when you look down and the hips move and when they don't. As you look down, can your hips begin sending the ball back immediately or does it take more time before the ball moves? What and where are the sensations and tensions?

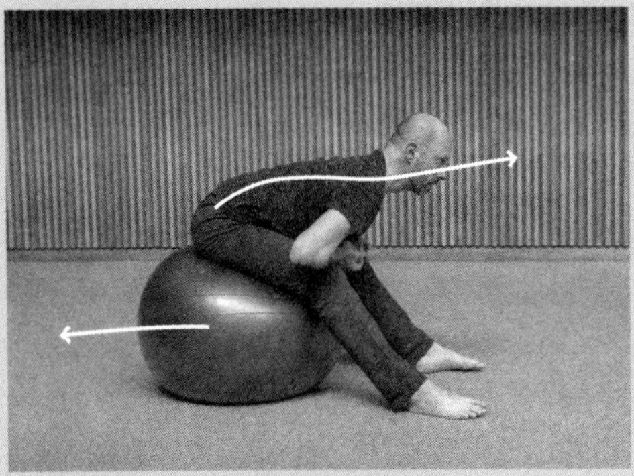

3. Secondary Ball Back or *looking at the ocean*: Give up the curling activity, letting the spine unfurl while continuing to move the ball back. The spine is long and the ball is about as far back as it can go. Make sure you maintain contact with the floor with both feet. Depending on the size of the ball and your height, your legs may still be somewhat bent or nearly straight. Notice that you can see the floor. During this phase, as the ball continues to go back, you can also look up, slightly out in front of you (to see the ocean) but not so far that you overly arch your neck or back. The overall pattern is an easy, long extension of the spine.

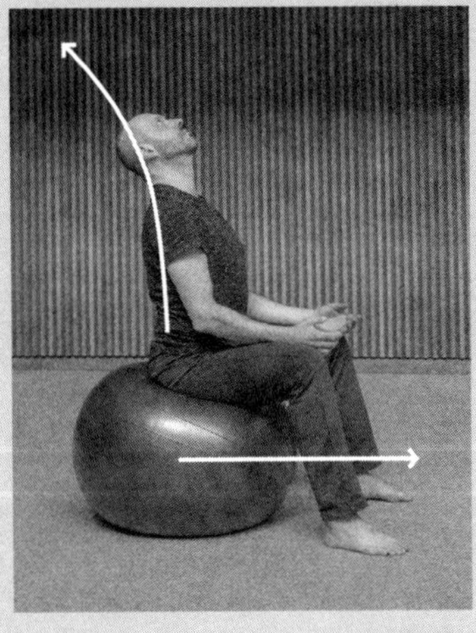

4. Secondary Ball Forward or *looking for seagulls*: Now that the ball is as far back as it can go and your spine is fully extended, begin to look up farther along the floor to the wall across from you and then toward the ceiling, allowing the whole torso to follow. Ideally, as soon as you look up, the ball should change direction and begin to move forward. As explored in Chapter Four, looking up is an integrated, whole-spine activity and does not require a huge arch in the neck or back. For movers who are used to experiencing more extreme movement, one can look very far up to engage an overall hyperextension in the spine, but always with *the ball going forward.*

From this last phase, return to Primary Ball Forward/*resting in the beach chair* by giving up the idea of extension/arch. Allow the ball to continue forward, soften the front body, and allow your gaze to Reset toward the horizon, returning to sitting back in your *beach chair.*

Here are a few things to keep in mind when exploring these Four Phases:

1. The amount or range of motion does not matter. These phases can be explored in a large range of motion or very subtly.
2. Do not try to force the ball's movement; it should move organically in response to the activity of the head and back. If you find that the ball does not automatically go in these directions when you try the sequences, play around more to explore your habits and tendencies.

3. Remember that the use of the legs and arms can hinder or help your ability to flow through these sequences; as we have explored in previous chapters, they are not neutral and can participate throughout the whole movement.
4. It is also important not to look for a clean separation between the phases. It is more appropriate to think of them as overlapping, so that as one phase is happening, the second is already entering a preparation phase, making itself available the moment it is needed.

Once comfortable with each phase, it is important to link them all together into one flowing, uninterrupted phrase. As you do this, pay special attention to interferences that disrupt the integration in the flow between phases. This allows you to notice your habitual preferences in activity. For example, the ball may get "stuck" and not move for a while when you look up or down. You might not enjoy the sensation of sending the ball forward when in Primary Ball Forward/*resting in the beach chair* or unintentionally send the ball back more as you start to look up. Getting acquainted with these moments of interference will help you see them in other more complex movement.

If you have access to a small inflatable ball (as mentioned in the Introduction to Part Three), you can explore these same movements in a smaller, more subtle way. Sit on a chair and place the ball right under your pelvic floor, so that your two ischial tuberosities, your coccyx, and your pubic bone are touching the ball. Do the same movements as above, allowing the ball to respond as before. In this case, you can experience the dynamic and responsive movements of the pelvis in relationship to the head, even though they may be quite small. These minute adjustments are key for maintaining flexibility and adaptability as we move.

Video: Animated Four Phases

Around when I was intensively writing my thesis paper, I began to experience a stiff and uncomfortable lower back. When I wasn't warm or had been sitting for long periods of time, I was having trouble performing simple activities such as bending over to tie my shoes. While certain stretching and strengthening activities recommended by a physical therapist were helpful, the Framework for Integration helped me to rethink how I was sitting. While I always thought that I should "sit up straight" while typing (meaning, largely in Secondary with an arched spine, ball back), I decided to try "slumping," which I previously believed to involve "bad" posture. As I typed, I thought about sending the ball forward and leaning back slightly, with a few extra pillows for support. This slight Primary greatly relieved the discomfort, as I inhibited my habit of sitting in Secondary.

—Sarah Mininsohn, Dance graduate student, University of Illinois

Arms and Legs in the Sagittal Plane

As you explore all these possibilities of the head and pelvis on the ball, it will not take you long to observe how supportive or interfering the limbs can be. Below is a simple way to explore the arms and legs in the traditional Four Phases that we just did in Movement Exploration 7.2.

MOVEMENT EXPLORATION 7.3: FOUR PHASES ADDING LIMB DIRECTIONS

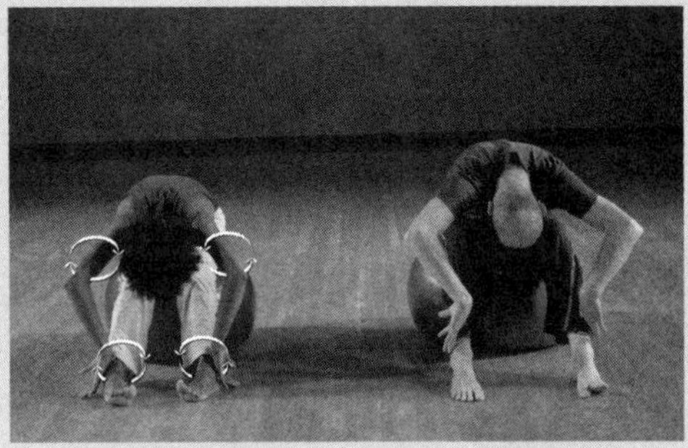

During the Primary Ball Forward phase (*Beach Chair*): With the ball going forward and generally looking toward the horizon, your arms will tend to move toward pronation (thumb side rotating in), and your legs/hips will tend to start going toward inward rotation (big toes pointing in).

During the Primary Ball Back phase (*Sandals*): As you look down, sending the ball back, with a slight bend of the elbows, the arms continue pronating. Meanwhile, the legs continue rotating inward as the ball escapes back.

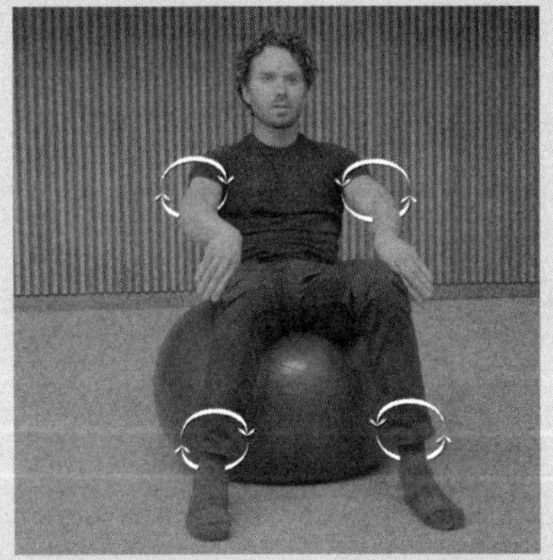

During the Secondary Ball Back phase (*Ocean*): As you start to extend your spine, the arms will start to move toward supination (palms facing up), and the legs will let go of their inward rotation as you send the ball back.

During the Secondary Ball Forward phase (*Seagulls*): As you start to look up and the ball changes direction to go forward, the arms continue to supinate while the legs move toward outward rotation.

Returning to Primary Ball Forward phase (*Beach Chair*): As you Reset your spine with the ball continuing to go forward, your arms will move toward pronation and your legs let go of the outward rotation.

Video: Four Phases Adding Limb Direction

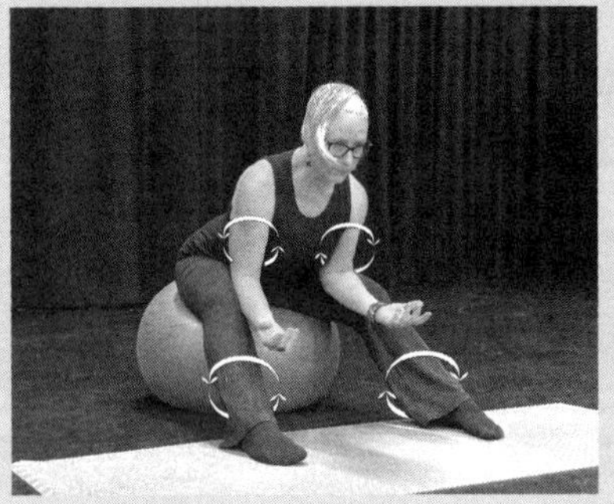

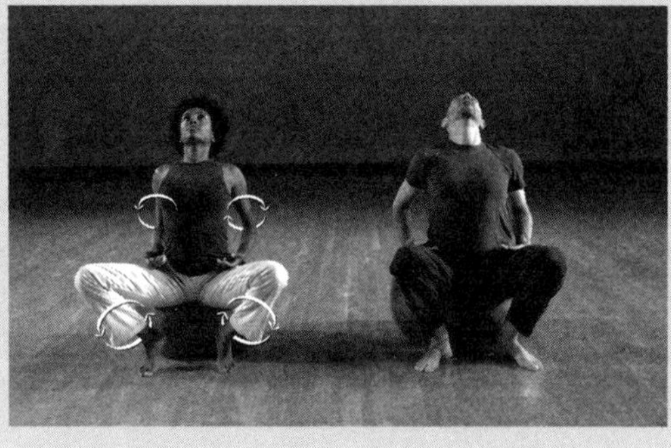

This cycle builds on our previous discussions of the limbs' relationship to the whole in the Simple and Complex Models. The limb directions in the Four Phases demonstrate how our limbs are or are not participating appropriately in the movement. Through exploring this work, you will discover that the underlying structures at play are more complex than you may have originally thought due to the underlying double-spiral arrangement. Throughout this chapter we have explored the double spirals symmetrically. The next step is to explore the Complex Model on the ball, where we will experience spirals asymmetrically.

Spirals on the Ball

In the Simple Model, we initially worked in the sagittal plane and then moved to spirals. The next step in exploring the ball mirrors that progression and now calls for three-dimensional spiraling. Strangely enough, we start spirals by moving side to side or laterally on the ball. The ideas for these explorations germinated in Luc and Jacklyn's research (see Introduction to Part Three). One particular thing Luc observed was how people in wheelchairs instinctively spiraled or angled themselves when speaking to someone who was standing. When a standing person was directly in front of them, the height difference often forced the person in the wheelchair to strain the neck to look up, a tiring demand on the person in lower spatial level. Often, the person in the wheelchair would maneuver the chair in a diagonal to the standing person and then shift his weight away from them in a counterspiral.

MOVEMENT EXPLORATION 7.4:
LATERAL WEIGHT SHIFTS ON THE BALL

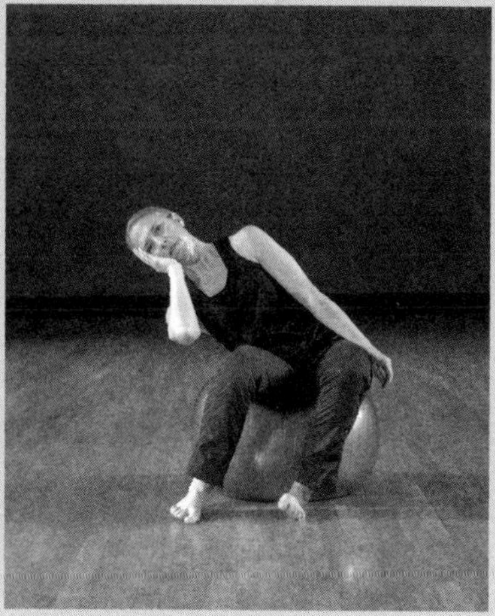

Begin by sitting on the ball. Bring your right hand to your right cheek. Apply pressure into the palm of your hand, keeping your torso connected as a whole while shifting your weight onto your right hip. See if the ball will escape left as your weight transfers more fully onto your right hip. In the Framework, our mantra is "spirals transfer weight," so even though this motion may look as if you are keeping your body flat in the frontal plane, the spirals of your body are actually facilitating the ball moving sideways.

Repeat this movement similarly, but this time also turn your head to the left while transferring your weight onto your right hip, actually leading the weight transfer with the back of your head (here, you can move your hand from your cheek to the back of your head for continued support—eyes direct upward).

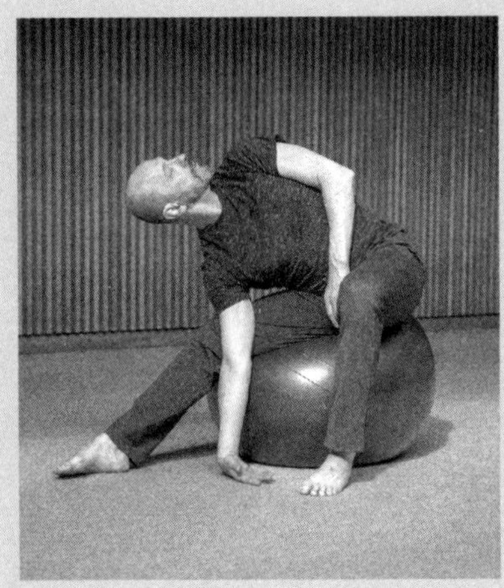

If you have already practiced your spirals, you will recognize the activity in your body: your right shoulder wants to go slightly forward and is getting freer the more your right hip connects to the ball (and the ball escapes to the left). The left hip is also getting freer and going toward leaving the ball; the left leg is Resetting (getting freer with the possibility of being able to lift the left foot off the floor). The left shoulder will open in Secondary. Looking again at the activity of the arms, the right arm is generally pronating (Primary) and the left arm is generally supinating (Secondary). The legs are doing something similar, with the right leg more toward turning out (Secondary) and the left leg more toward turning in (Primary). This particular movement exercise requires that the opposing spirals come into coordinated play. Try it on the other side. Did you notice specific differences or interferences?

The immediacy of staying balanced on the ball allows us to recognize interferences in the ways we approach our spirals. Differences are likely in the ways we undertake and experience each side. Asymmetries are especially noticeable when doing this kind of spiraling and are present in nearly everything we do. The goal here is not to work toward perfect anatomical balance or symmetry. Except for truly ambidextrous individuals, most people are one-side dominant in most daily routines and activities. With an understanding of spirals, we can bring conscious awareness to approaches and patterns that interfere with or unnecessarily complicate what we intend to do. Also, in many movement activities, we tend to "flatten out" our spirals by capitulating to faulty ideas of structural strength and symmetry. Through these spiraling explorations on the ball, we hope that you will begin to recognize where you can enhance the natural spirals in your movement. Spirals on the ball facilitate a needed transference of knowledge that can apply to more complex movement (such as walking, running, swimming, and yoga practice).

Now that you have spiraled from side to side, experiencing the Engaging, freeing, and Resetting of the hips and legs, it is time to play with spiraling and weight shifting even more.

MOVEMENT EXPLORATION 7.5: CIRCLING

Part One: Circling to the Front

Once again, transfer your weight to the right while turning your head to the left. Now, change your gaze by turning your nose/eyes slowly toward the floor while also moving the ball backward in space until you are in a Primary Ball Back (*Sandals*). In other words, your torso will lean sideways and then roll forward as the ball goes back. Next, turn your head toward the right, shifting your weight to the left hip, continuing to move the ball to the right. To finish, Reset your gaze forward to let the hips guide the ball back to its original starting point.

Part Two: Circling to the Back

Now let's go the opposite way. Transferring your weight to the right while turning your head to the left, let your nose/eyes turn toward the ceiling as the ball escapes forward in space until you are in a Secondary Ball Forward (*Seagulls*). Then, looking up and over to your right, feel the ball start to make its way toward the right as your weight shifts to the left hip. Finally, let the hips guide the ball back to its original starting point with your head facing forward.

Part Three: Putting the Two Together: Full Circle

Let's do Part One into Part Two. As in Part One, transfer your weight to the right while turning your head to the left. Then change your gaze by turning your nose/eyes toward the floor while also moving the ball backward until you are in a Primary Ball Back (*Sandals*). Then, turn your head toward the right as the ball also continues right, shifting your weight to your left hip. Right away, continue in the opposite way (Part Two), transferring your weight to both hips as you look up toward the ceiling, the ball escaping forward to arrive in Secondary Ball Forward (*Seagulls*). Looking up and over to your left, feel the ball start to make its way toward the left as your weight shifts to the right hip and then let the hips guide the ball back to its original starting point facing forward.

Video: Circling

This movement exercise could be continuous, creating multiple circles built from these spirals. These explorations are meant primarily to find the moments when we are less comfortable, interfering, or habitually locking (stopping the ball from moving). These are not necessarily exercises that need to be repeated over and over as skill building—at least not without a clear, directed understanding of what we are looking to inhibit or allow. We encourage you to explore these spirals on the ball in parts or whole, looping, pausing, or reversing according to what interests you.

Once you have some familiarity with the ball and these explorations, you can begin to consider where your imaginary *ball* is going in your daily routines and activities. Where is your *ball* going when you brush your teeth or wash dishes? Does it need to go in that direction, or can you play with other choices? Can you include thoughts of *ball* direction while you are driving, walking, or going up and down stairs? Throughout the remainder of the book, we will include these *ball* directions.

> Throughout the semester, what has stuck with me the most has been the movement of the "ball." Which way the head is positioned affects how the pelvis moves. Even though it seems like such a simple concept, I wonder how I ever moved before. I have seen it translate to the rest of my classes. Furthermore, I have begun to learn where my "head" is instead of my face. Feeling that for the first time was a wild sensation. This is a feeling I hope I can remember as my time here progresses.
>
> —Liz Connor, Dance undergraduate student, University of Florida

Chapter 8

Upper and Lower Triangles

The Observation of Upper and Lower Triangles and Their Antagonistic Action[1]

> **Increasing consciousness = Increasing Complexity**
>
> **—Ken Wilber, *A Theory of Everything***

As noted previously, the work on the ball eventually reveals an increasing complexity. In earlier models of the ball work, we identified Primary Ball Forward as a whole-body activity in Primary. But after working with the model in Alexander teacher training, we eventually assessed that upper and lower trunk actions were different, especially in terms of Engagements and Resets. Moving through the Four Phases, there clearly were varying distributions of muscular effort needed to move the ball while also staying balanced. We noticed that Engagements and Resets met and overlapped in various places in the body, and in these areas of overlap, stability and mobility intersected, especially at the top of the spine, which related to the head and neck being able to free up as well as support movement intention overall. This most recent lens in the Framework delineates the double-spiral musculature through two overlapping triangles. These ideas were influenced by observations that Luc made while conducting research on equine rehabilitation at Postural Rehabilitation for horses and dogs in Nottingham, Pennsylvania. What he learned from watching AT teachers and vets encouraging horses to shift weight between upper and lower limbs (for shoeing and repatterning, for example) germinated into what we have now translated as these triangles for bipedal humans.

As Alexander Technique teachers, we honor the concept of *Primary Control,* which refers to the head's coordination in relationship to the rest of the spine. What are the various complex synergies at play that allow the "head to lead and the body to follow"? We know that horses can easily be led by their halter—only their teeth and jaws need to be directed for the head and whole body to follow suit.

MOVEMENT EXPLORATION 8.1:
PRIMARY CONTROL ILLUSTRATION LYING PRONE

Lie prone with your forehead touching the floor, elbows bent and forearms along the floor. Now, leaving your head down, try to pull yourself forward along the floor. You will probably find it almost impossible to move forward, or if you are managing to move, you are using an inordinate amount of effort in the shoulders and back to make it happen. Now look forward and up to see something in front of you, and try again to pull yourself forward, making sure your elbows stay down. This should be easier and more coordinated. Even just the thought of lifting the head will help facilitate the movement.

Video: Primary Control Illustration Lying Prone

Notice it takes the whole body to raise the head. This can be seen clearly in an alligator rising off the ground to crawl. The head leads, the legs push, and the back comes up and back in a Primary. Clearly some effort toward the floor is needed to allow the rest of the body to extend itself, in this case a push in Primary. This is an unmistakable example of antagonistic action—this principle (refer to Chapter Three: Infrastructure) also supports the process of coming all the way to standing. The Framework aims to clarify this concept as we seek to understand the antagonistic action involved in overall coordinated functioning.

MOVEMENT EXPLORATION 8.2:
ROCKING BACK AND FORTH ON ALL FOURS

Another place to explore is on the floor on hands and knees, feeling the weight equally on all fours. An adapted standing version would be to lean over with your hands on the seat of a chair, supporting your upper body weight. Now, slowly look up and allow the looking to transfer your weight onto your hands. You might notice that while your hands are receiving more weight, your knees may be able to release, easing their amount of support from the floor (can you wobble and wiggle your hips, knees, and legs?). Now, let your head Reset and allow the weight to naturally transfer backward toward your knees/feet. As you feel your weight transfer back through your pelvis and knees/legs to your feet, start to notice that your hands now feel very little weight against the floor/chair—your lower body is supporting more of your torso's weight. Any child or animal does this (we see this rocking between the upper and lower body explicitly in babies getting ready to crawl), but what we find fascinating is the *activity of the head/neck/spine in relationship to the limbs* as we move back and forth between our knees/feet and hands. As you come forward and your hands are engaged against the floor/chair, can you feel your neck Resetting (perhaps freer) in opposition to that Engagement? And as you move backward, can you feel your head/neck reorganize into Engagement (perhaps a feeling of strength) as your arms Reset? In moving forward and back between the support from your arms and legs, notice changes in the tone of your neck.

Video: Rocking Back and Forth on All Fours

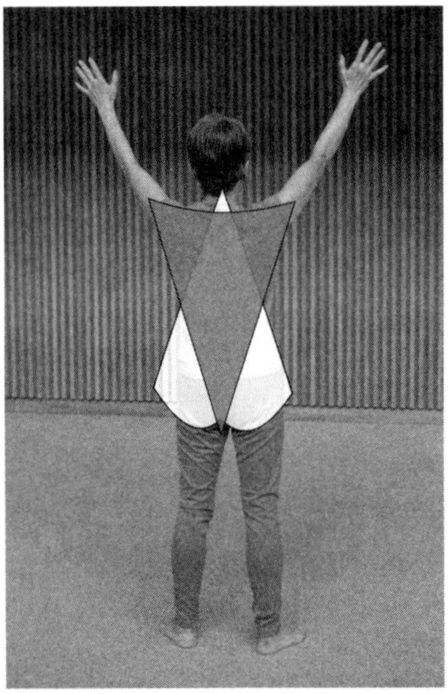

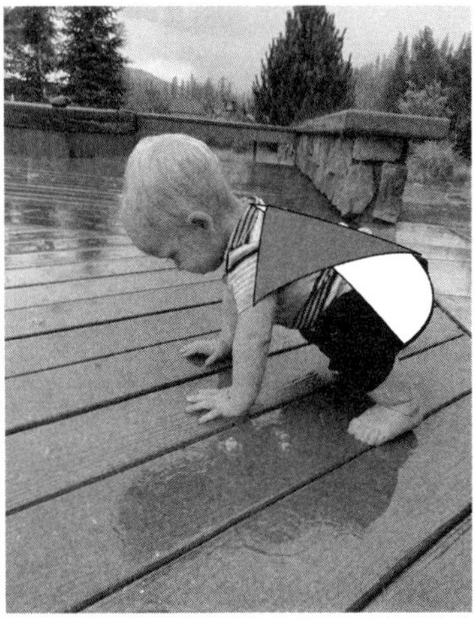

Oppositional Connections: Upper and Lower Triangles

A simple image to introduce this concept is a turtle stuck on its back that uses its head to look for support to bring itself back on its legs: One double spiral works against the other. It is also relatively easy to see in a sitting or standing dog or horse. The neck is looking to extend itself while the legs are reaching or pushing against the ground. It is also possible to observe in a bird flapping its wings downward while extending its neck in the direction of flight. We propose that one action cannot exist without the other—pushing down without extending is not typical in the movement of animals and children. This push-while-extending coordination is a direct result of the double-spiral musculature.

These animal and developmental movement examples and images inspired us to superimpose imaginary triangles on the body so we could observe the upper and lower body activity coordinated through opposition. The wide base of the "upper" triangle is drawn across the back and shoulders and narrows down to the sacrum/coccyx. The "lower" triangle originates in a wide base across the bottom of the pelvis and extends all the way up to the occipital ridge. Looking at the accompanying photo, pay special attention to the areas where each triangle's point emerges from underneath the opposite triangle's base. These overlaps create a strength built by opposition, often Engagement against Reset, and Primary against Secondary intents.

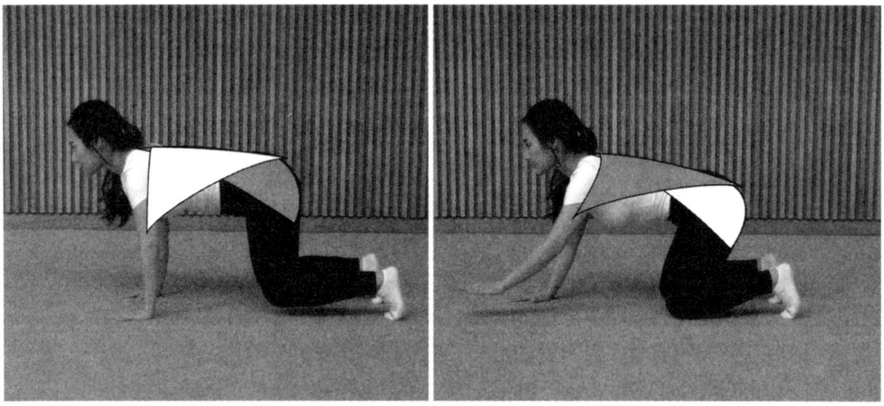

MOVEMENT EXPLORATION 8.3: HANDS CROSSING AT WRISTS

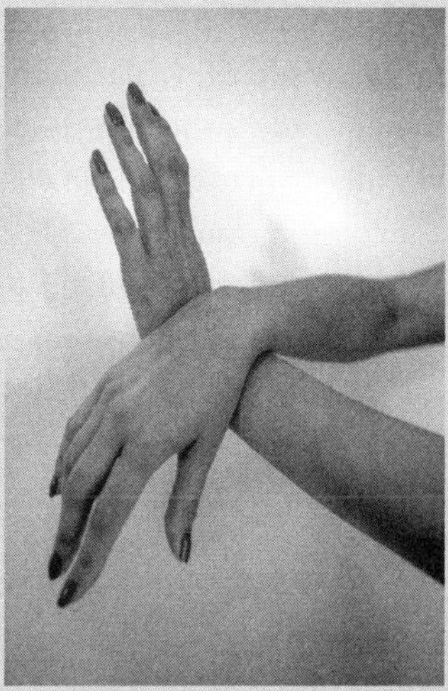

We can represent this opposition with our hands crossing at both wrists to demonstrate the two interlocking intents. Cross one hand over the other at the wrist. The bottom hand represents the upper triangle while the top hand represents the lower triangle. Notice also that the bottom hand is active in Secondary and the top is Resetting in Primary. One Engages while the other Resets. Feel the connection at the junction. It might be possible to do double Primary and/or double Secondary with your hands, but feel how unsupportive this is to the connection between both wrists.

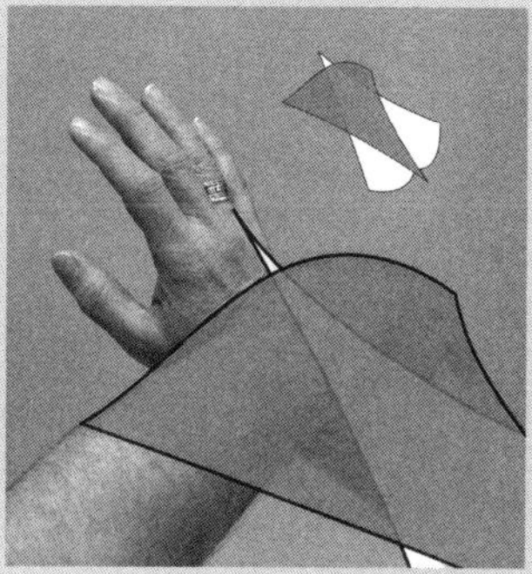

The next exploration allows us to see the opposition in our own backs and limbs.

MOVEMENT EXPLORATION 8.4: CRAWLING ON ALL FOURS REVISITED: UPPER AND LOWER TRIANGLES

Return to the floor on hands and knees or the standing alternative with the chair. Again, look up and allow the looking to transfer your weight onto your hands. This is Engaging your Upper Triangle and Resetting your Lower Triangle. Now, let your head Reset and allow the weight to naturally transfer backward toward your knees or feet. This is Engaging your Lower Triangle and Resetting your Upper Triangle. Notice the overlapping phrasing of Engagements and Resets.

Video: Crawling on All Fours Revisited: Upper and Lower Triangles

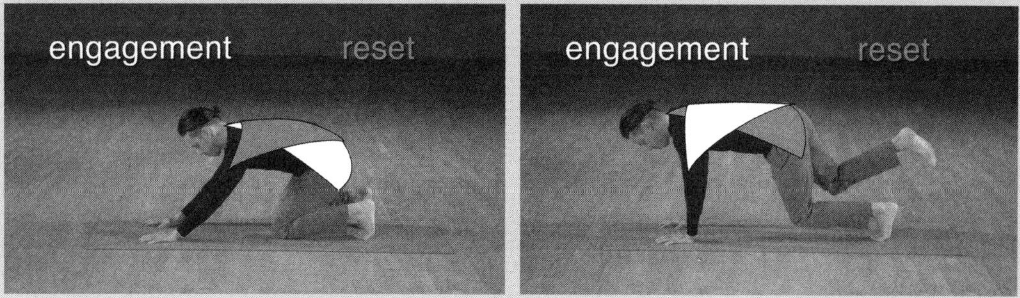

Another application we find useful, in working with Upper and Lower Triangles and antagonistic action, is how to reorganize the bodily patterning needed to do a squat. Most able-bodied toddlers squat easily and frequently—squatting is an inherent, organic action in the lexicon of movement skills we master early in life. The next time you see a toddler busily exploring all the curiosities and levels of her environment, notice how many times she effortlessly lowers and rises from squatting (even with such a big head!). Most of the populace around the globe squats as a matter of daily activity, and many animals such as squirrels, dogs, and primates comfortably allow their hind quarters to reach the floor to rest. Squats represent an extreme range of the mix of mobility, stability, coordination, and skill needed to do what might be considered the "adult" task of sitting down in a chair, and from the whole body, not just the hips, knees, and ankles. Soon after this stage of childhood, as we imitate our older siblings and adults, sitting on chairs and couches and being generally inactive, our modern Western bodies quickly forget this birthright.

The movement exploration below features one of many ways to approach squatting. Adapt everything as needed, and if the joint range of motion feels too extreme, tense, or painful in any part of your body (neck, back, and knees especially), these explorations can be left for another day. In training Alexander Technique teachers, we have found that by employing the Framework principles gently over time, people who believed they could never achieve a squat, now with coordination and confidence lower and rise from squats with smiles on their faces!

MOVEMENT EXPLORATION 8.5: SQUATTING WITH A CHAIR

First, stand upright, feet wide and apart, facing a chair with a back that will allow you to walk your hands down its sides or back. Use a light chair on a nonskid surface such as a yoga mat. During this exploration, it might be necessary to keep widening your stance.

1. Put your hands on the top of the back of the chair and start slowly tilting the chair forward onto two legs.
2. Similar to Movement Exploration 8.4, transfer your weight onto your hands as you push the chair. This will free up your legs as they stay away in the opposite direction of the push.

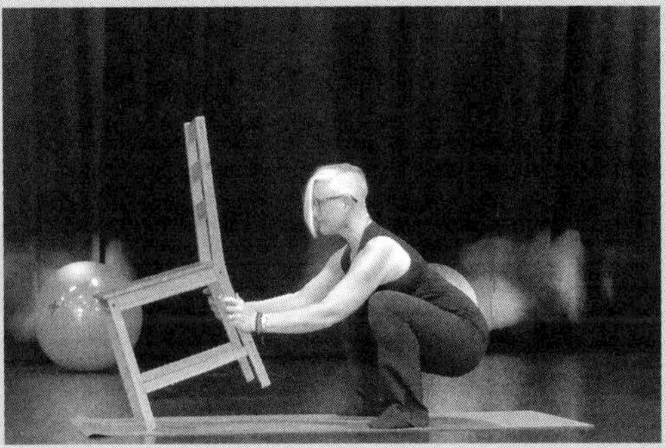

3. Use the Reset to let your legs bend a little (include awareness of ankles, knees, and hips) and then transfer your weight onto them without adding too much pressure. Watch for the habit of wanting to push your weight down into your legs.
4. Then repeat the process of transferring your weight forward and back (with the push of the chair), each time releasing your knees more and then reaching farther out in space with the push of the chair. This back and forth will bring you lower and lower until you

need to start walking your hands down the back/sides of the chair, tipping the chair more and more forward and eventually even walking your hands down its legs.

5. You are going toward a full squat to end up in a deep Primary with your arms reaching forward (the chair may end up tipping way over). The pelvis is between your feet (which may need to widen), Resetting all the way to your tail (note: Resetting the tail is not tucking the tail).

6. In the squat, feel the balance wanting to shift between the push and pull of the arms/Upper and Lower Triangles. Notice whether one triangle might want to take over too strongly. If you feel too much stress in the legs, Engage a pull to your arms. Or see if a push of the arms will keep your spine supported and can help your pelvis stay buoyant.

7. Then, letting yourself Reset forward, reverse the process, climbing up the back of the chair, slightly rocking forward and back and then up to standing.

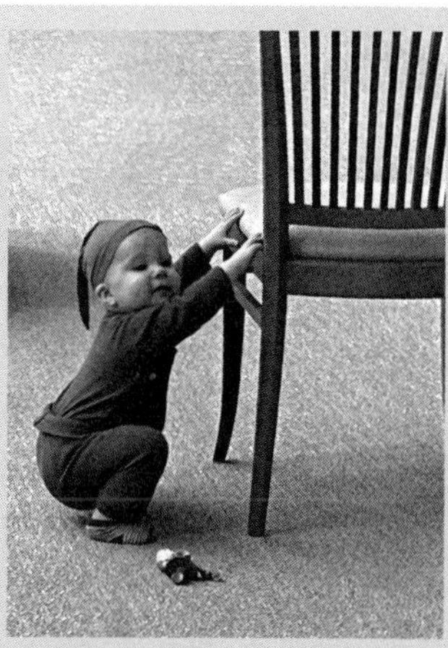

Video: Squatting with a Chair

Things to think about:

The activity of tilting the chair forward is designed to free the legs and hips. If you find yourself struggling or falling forward, it's your hips trying to push the chair and not your hands. Readjust by allowing the natural opposition of your hips (*ball* back) as arms reach away. Do not force the bending of your legs in this exploration. If being in deep flexion is not appropriate for you at this time, consider adding a stool, physioball, yoga blocks, or bolster to sit on as you get lower toward squatting. Slowly lower the height of any aids/props as you gain more mobility and confidence.

The antagonistic action present in these movement explorations can also be seen on the ball. Having introduced the triangles, we will now revisit our Four Phases model in relationship to the Upper and Lower Triangles in the following chapter.

NOTE

1. At this moment, "triangles" remain the clearest descriptor we have found for these organizational structures, though "cones" has also been considered. Each term has limitations. Triangles can sound overly rigid and geometric, while cones better suggest curvature but still fail to fully convey the flexibility and responsiveness of the living body. Our original conception of the triangles was always meant to imply curved, adaptable structures wrapping through the body more like portions of cones than fixed flat planes. As you read, keep in mind that these terms are approximations meant to point toward dynamic relationships in action rather than static shapes.

Chapter 9

Circling Back: Triangles in Weight Shifting, Ball Work, and Spirals

Now that the Upper and Lower Triangles have been introduced, we can circle back to include and apply this awareness to the Simple and Complex Models. Try layering the triangles into previous movement explorations. This lens adds further detail to understanding weight shifting in sitting, standing, and the Four Phases on the ball.

By now, through practicing the movement explorations, it has likely become increasingly apparent how movable the pelvis actually is—a crucial factor in the moment-by-moment processes of movement and balance. The experience on the ball provides applied spatial support and focus, rather than trying to control balance and movement directly through shape or "correct" muscularized posture or alignment. We now reframe all the elements of coordinated movement through this lens by asking, "Where is the imaginary *ball* going?" even as orientation in space and posture change. Understanding that the *ball* is always there and moving, even when we are standing, has been revolutionary in our approach to teaching movement skills.

The art of simplicity is a puzzle of complexity.

—Douglas Horton (attributed)

Transferring our weight in standing, which leads to walking and running, is a prime example of the complexity of timing Engagements and Resets. The *ball* moves, one side Engages, and one side Resets. The head or the hips can lead or follow—there is no right way—but the sequencing can clarify profoundly how we are coordinating ourselves in fundamental, necessary, and ubiquitous movements. Circling back to previous movement explorations, we start again on the ball and then move to standing weight shifts.

Though the Four Phases were originally anchored in Primary and Secondary, layering in the Upper and Lower Triangles clarifies what parts of the body are actually Engaging and Resetting.

MOVEMENT EXPLORATION 9.1: UPPER AND LOWER TRIANGLES IN THE FOUR PHASES ON THE BALL

Starting in Primary Ball Forward (*Beach Chair*), see if you can notice the Upper Triangle being Engaged while the lower is Resetting. This relates to being on all fours with your weight transferred onto your hands and arms. If you have a partner who can help you by putting a hand on your upper back, it is even easier to notice how the Upper Triangle Engages. Sitting far back on the ball with it directing forward, you can feel the muscular strength of the trunk flexors stabilizing you, but you also may be able to notice that your pelvis, legs, and feet are Reset (freer than the upper). In the wild, a bear might find support to scratch their upper back on a tree with the pelvis forward and legs free.

Video: Primary Ball Forward (Beach Chair) with partner

As we transition to another phase in Primary Ball Back (*Sandals*), we see this balance between the upper and lower body shift; as the torso goes forward and the ball changes in direction, the strength and push of the legs takes over, allowing the Upper Triangle to Reset. Keep in mind that no effort should be made to come forward with the head or the upper trunk in the transition from Primary Ball Forward to Primary Ball Back. Instead, thinking of coming "up and back" on an upbeat and then over will help you direct the ball backward in space. The only way to do this is to coordinate your legs with your trunk—another way of saying that the Lower Triangle is being activated or Engaged. On the web, it's easy to find fun videos of pandas doing forward rolls with their hips continually being tossed up in the air.

Video: Primary Ball Back (Sandals) with partner

The exchange between Upper and Lower Engaging and Resetting is also apparent in Secondary Ball Back (*Ocean*) and Secondary Ball Forward (*Seagulls*). When the ball goes back in Secondary, the Upper Triangle supports and the Lower Triangle Resets. This might be the clearest correlation of our previous exploration on all fours in Movement Exploration 8.2. We could liken this action to a horse extending forward on forelegs to kick back in space.

From Secondary Ball Back, at the very moment where your interest in looking up becomes strong enough to move the ball forward, you transition fully into Secondary Ball Forward, with the Lower Triangle of the legs and pelvis powering the extension with the Upper Triangle Resetting. That moment is similar to a horse rearing on its hind legs.

Now we can add this awareness and vocabulary to the Four Phases:

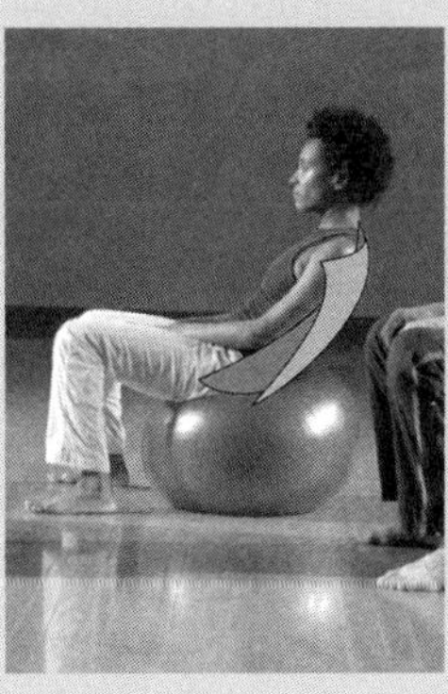

1. Primary ball forward (*Beach Chair*) = Upper Triangle Engaged and Lower Triangle Reset

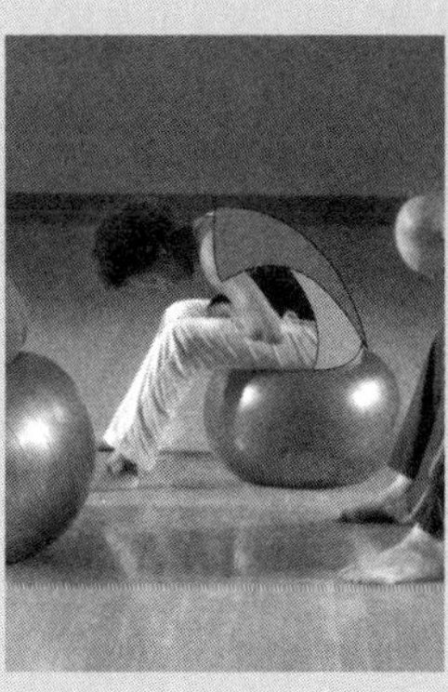

2. Primary ball back (*Sandals*) = Lower Triangle Engaged and Upper Triangle Reset

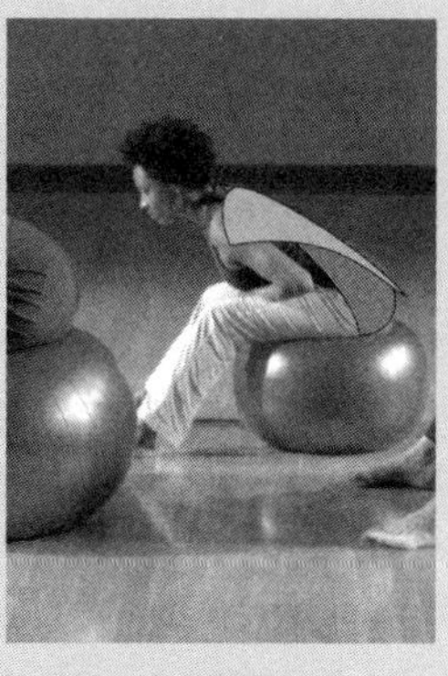

3. Secondary ball back (*Ocean*) = Upper Triangle Engaged and Lower Triangle Reset

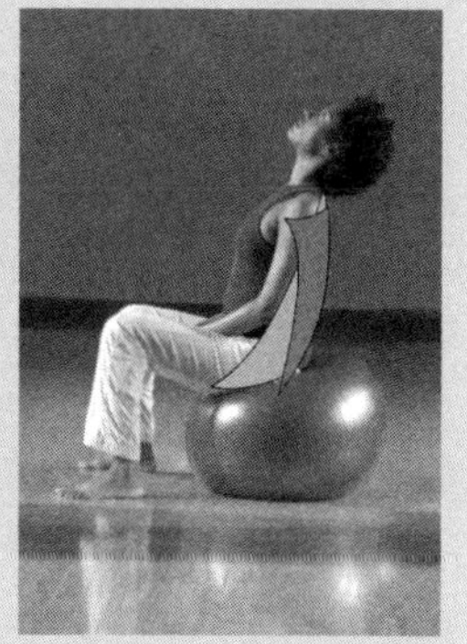

4. Secondary ball forward (*Seagulls*) = Lower Triangle Engaged and Upper Triangle Reset

Here are a few things to keep in mind when exploring the Four Phases with Upper and Lower Triangle Engagements and Resets:

1. An *Engagement* of the Lower Triangle will always change the ball's direction through the action of the pelvis.
2. A *Reset* of the Lower Triangle will always continue the ball in the direction you were already going.
3. *The ball moves as soon as the thought initiates the action.*
4. By nature, we are not perfectly symmetrical beings. We prefer certain phases over others, certain triangles, and certain sides of the triangles.

Once you can see these upper and lower exchanges of support at play, it is hard to dismiss them, especially in animals such as a rearing horse or a sprinting cheetah. If the complexity of this activity feels like a lot to add to your awareness, continuing to explore the original Four Phases should eventually lend itself to understanding more about the Upper and Lower Engagements and Resets.

This addition of Upper and Lower Triangles helps us clarify how it "feels" to work with Engagements and Resets on the ball. Depending on habits and movement preferences, some phases may feel more muscularly arduous in some places. Using the triangles to assess what might be the most efficient and organic transfers of weight and support can help us let go of overly activating our entire musculature.

Here are some examples of Upper and Lower Triangle exchanges on the ball:

- Pulling on a yoga strap held by a partner standing in front of you as you send the ball back helps release the hip joints (*Ocean*—an Upper Engagement helps Reset the Lower Triangle).
- Putting your head in your hands, as if crying, while sending the ball forward, will help free the pelvis and release the legs (*Beach Chair*—an Upper Engagement helps Reset the Lower Triangle).
- Putting the hands together in prayer also encourages an Upper Engagement that can free the legs, whether we are looking up (*Seagulls*—with ball forward while the hands pull to the elbow) or down (*Sandals*—with ball back while the hands are pushing).

You can now ask yourself questions like: When I am looking up in Secondary Ball Forward, do I need all this tension in my arms? Do I have *enough* tension when in Secondary Ball Back? When weight and support are exchanging, what is going on in my head/neck—do I need more support or freedom right now?

These questions are especially relevant when considering squatting. Here, we revisit the squat we did in Chapter Eight but now integrate the Four Phases on the ball with Upper and Lower Triangles.

MOVEMENT EXPLORATION 9.2: SQUATTING REVISITED

Stand tall with your feet slightly apart. While standing, consider where your *ball* wants to go habitually.

1. Directing the *ball* back (hips), incline yourself forward in space.
2. Let your head reach over toward the floor, hands reaching to the floor as you now direct the *ball* to the ceiling, sending your hips up. This is a *Sandals* phase and looks akin to "forward fold" in a yoga practice. If you cannot yet reach the floor with your hands, feel free to use your hands on your legs (other supports could be a low stool or yoga blocks).
3. Start to look up along the floor as if someone in front of you called your name. On whatever surface your hands and arms are supported, they change from a natural push to a pull (notice if you don't want to include your arms, and loop back to do so if you weren't). While continuing to pull (Upper Triangle Engagement), allow yourself to come to an *Ocean* phase with the *ball* still going back and knees slightly bending, but now lengthening your spine as fully as possible. The legs and pelvis are free and bouncy. Notice if any part is working too hard (especially your neck) and see if you can distribute the Secondary extension throughout the whole spine.
4. Now continue looking up toward the ceiling (*Seagull* phase). Your legs will continue into deeper bending, and your *ball* will start to go forward. Keep going as far as you can, with your hips lowering to a squat between your feet—you can look up all the way to the ceiling if possible. The Engagement is now in the legs.
5. Let go of this Engaged spinal extension and allow yourself to Reset in a Primary Ball Forward (*Beach Chair*), Resetting the head on top, which may feel like looking down or lowering the chin toward the chest. Stay there for a moment and breathe. The Engagement is now in the Upper.
6. To start to get out of the squat, look down, sending your hips back up in the air (*ball* back) as you send the top of your head down toward the floor. You are in a *Sandals* phase.
7. Look up as you pull with your arms and allow the *ball* (and hips) to continue backward in space. You are in an *Ocean* phase and the Engagement is in the Upper Triangle.
8. Transition into a *Seagulls* phase, let the weight transfer fully into the legs, and come up to standing while looking up along the wall in front of you all the way to the ceiling.
9. Let it all go and end up more in a *Beach Chair* phase, allowing your legs to feel free under you. Note that you don't have to lock your knees to come back to standing—they can be Reset, soft, and available.

Video: Squatting Revisited with Triangle Animation

As this version does not use the support of a prop, observing what range of motion is best for you is important. All these phases can be done in smaller range or with the assistance of props. Consider what might be helpful to you. Do you need something that will support your Primary, such as a chair, stool, yoga blocks, blankets, or bolster to help with pushing with the arms to find stability? Or do you need help with Secondary, using anchors that will help you pull at critical times, such as a doorknob, a table leg, or a ballet barre? Notice that first, before the pelvis lowers into a squat, there is a direction in the hips that is up and away from the floor. Coordinating the looking up with the squatting can be very organizing. The eyes and looking organize our intent or reason for doing something. That's why children squat; they have clear intentions! A squat happens as a result of the balance of Engagements and Resets in the whole body. This is something you have done before and can learn to do again. Take your time.

Spiral on Ball: Translation to Standing with Weight Shifting to Engage and Reset the Limbs

As we continue to explore spirals, we now add the Upper and Lower Triangles but with the caveat that we can look at them through halves of the body. Moving out of symmetry, for example initiating movement with our dominant side, we can start to imagine what *one side* of an Upper or Lower Triangle is doing (Engaging or Resetting). The exploration below helps elucidate this idea.

MOVEMENT EXPLORATION 9.3: SPIRALS IN TRANSFERRING WEIGHT WHILE STANDING

From standing, raise your right hand to your right cheek (similar to Movement Exploration 7.4 on the ball) and then, applying slight pressure into your hand, transfer your weight over the right leg, allowing your imaginary *ball* to move to the left. What happened to your left hip and leg? Is your left foot still trying to touch the floor evenly? Let your left leg Reset, free up, and leave the floor. Notice your arms—is the left freer than the right? Can it float up to the side? Touching your cheek helps you feel the Engagement of your right arm/shoulder girdle. In contrast, your left shoulder is Resetting/freeing up along with the left hip and leg. When you are ready to be done, allow the left hip to lead you back to standing on two feet.

Notice in the following video of a squatting baby the ease with which they switch their weight from side to side.

Video: Baby in Squat Doing Lateral Shifts

Now, with hands on both cheeks, repeat the weight transfer onto your right foot, but this time, as you return to fully upright, instead of initiating with the hip, explore leading with your head to come back to two feet (in a righting action). Feel how you use one hand to guide the weight transfer and the other hand to guide coming back to balance (and then loop to the other side in a small figure-eight action).

Video: Spirals in Transferring Weight While Standing

Do you prefer coming back to standing with the hip or the head? While neither is right or wrong, if either the pelvis or the head habitually takes over when weight shifting, there may be interferences to smooth coordination. Notice whether you are anticipating and overly activating the righting reflex.[1] At times, like when throwing a ball, it is important for the hip to lead the activity and then have the arms finish. In other cases, such as when skiing or riding a bike, having the head lead is more appropriate than the hips.

When out of integration with the spirals and the pelvis's movement, the righting reflex can cause interferences in coordinated walking, in the same way that the notion of a neutral pelvis may interfere with balancing and adapting the whole spine. If you are struggling with this exercise, try sitting on a chair where it's easier to feel the weight transfer from one ischial tuberosity to the other. Keep in mind that we are looking at what interferences arise in the activity more than trying to control it directly.

One place to practice this safely is on the floor, playing around like a toddler. The righting reflex is much less likely to interfere incorrectly when there is no danger of falling. In looking to explore spirals on the floor, we combined the ball work with triangle work and created four spiral rolls on the floor, starting either from lying on our backs or our fronts.

These are further described in the following videos.

Video: Spiraling on the Floor with Illustrated Ball Direction

In watching these videos, it is important to remember that Engagements and Resets work antagonistically throughout the body. As we start to see the oppositions at play between the Upper and Lower Triangles, eventually it is possible to notice a similar interaction between the right and left sides of the same triangle and start to marvel at their interaction with the other triangle in simple actions like walking or skating.

Video: Triangle Engagement and Reset While Rollerblading

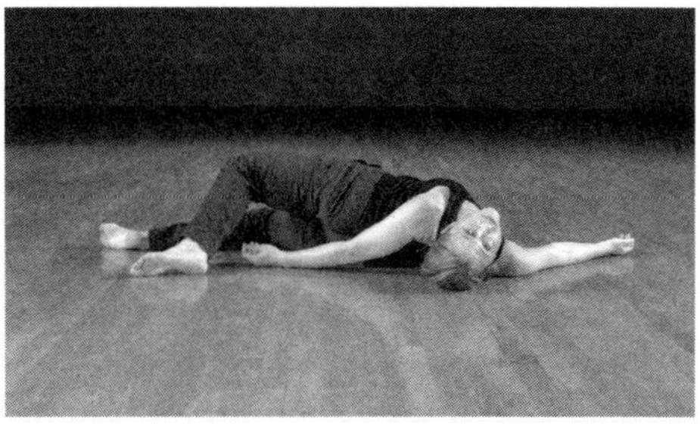

Rolling from supine to prone with a Secondary initiation

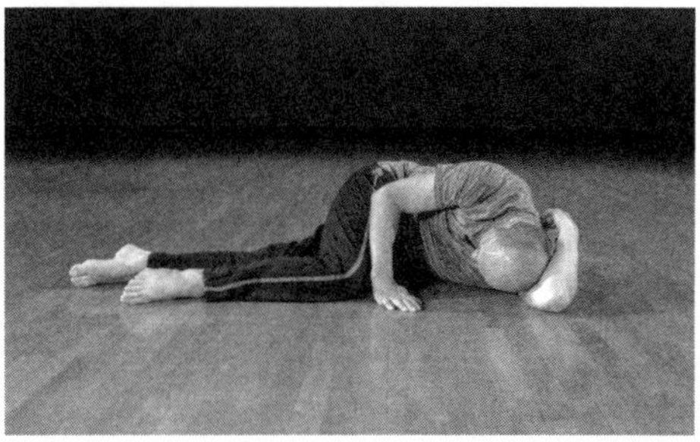

Rolling from prone to supine with a Primary initiation

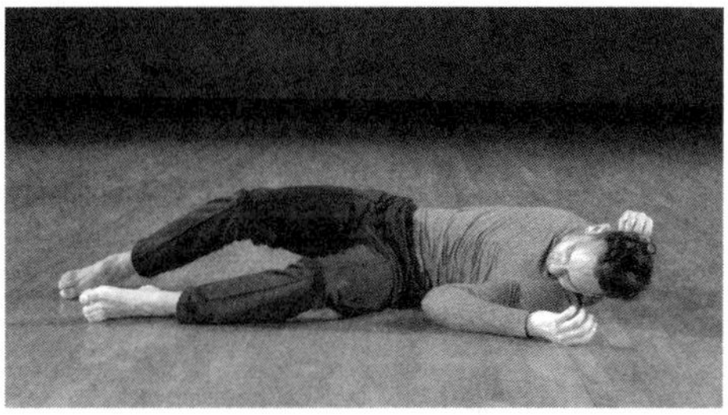

Rolling from supine to prone with a Primary initiation

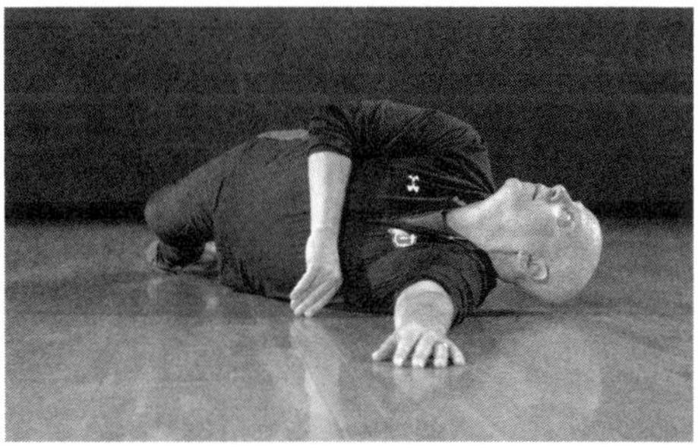

Rolling from prone to supine with a Secondary initiation

When It All Works

One of the more exciting discoveries about the Framework is the capacity of rhythm to provide feedback on our overall use. For example, learning how to move through the Four Phases on the ball becomes easier when there is clear rhythmic phrasing and transition, which is unique to each individual. Explore your tendencies and see what helps coordinate your movement. There is no objective, ideal rhythm; sometimes we think that evening out or containing the rhythm will help us control movement. It is common to find that fluidity is interrupted when the glitches of our unconscious preferences and habits show up. Such feedback is useful for redirecting interferences by observing which phase is being blocked or prematurely anticipated, and it can be of great help to movers and movement coaches alike. Also, noticing that our limbs tend to take on unnecessary responsibilities and tension not appropriate to their function can help us redirect our whole body with inhibitory thinking and the appropriate energy needed moment to moment, movement to movement.

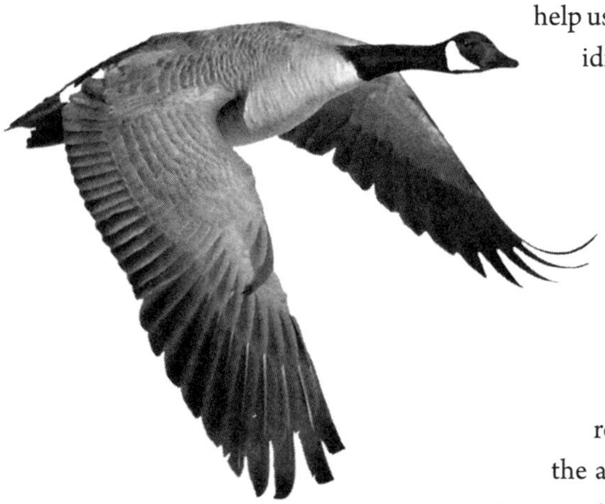

NOTE

1. The righting reflex in this case refers to the Labyrinthine Head Righting Reflex (LHRR). This reflex is responsible for maintaining the head in a vertical orientation in space, with eyes facing forward and level with the ears.

Part Four

Synthesis

Introduction

As you have made your way through the varied models and lenses of Framework for Integration, we hope you have engaged with the material lightly and playfully. We intend for this work to offer structures and tools for observing tendencies and preferences and also to provide a broader range of options and choices. We encourage toggling back and forth between recognizing when habits and propensities are useful and when they are not serving us. The transfer of information across all models is important, as is seeing how your sense of development as a mover and person is connected in all areas of your life. Bringing the relationship of the parts and the whole together and recognizing how the recurrent threads in the Framework models weave together in identifiable patterns equals synthesis.

In our work, supporting layered, developmental, effective learning can fuel curiosity and desire for ongoing growth and change. The process of changing can be a complicated affair. Attempts at changing even the simplest things in our lives often backfire, and superficial change is neither satisfying nor lasting. The word "change" implies shift, transformation, and difference from what was to what is to what might or will be. Being born into this world guarantees that, as the Greek philosopher Heraclitus opined in 535 BC, we will experience that "Change is the only constant in life." Our bodies reflect this radical truth from infancy to childhood, childhood to adolescence, adolescence to adulthood, middle age to old age. The human condition is to have the capacity to envision transformative change while simultaneously resisting it.

Chapter Ten, the Challenge of Change, discusses how working with the Framework supports greater, ongoing developmental change. Even when change is desired, interferences like deeply ingrained habits and echoes of trauma may arise and need to be addressed. Chapter Eleven zooms in to consider the Framework's applications to one of the most habitual, unconscious, and perhaps most intimate bodily processes: breathing. Once the overarching patterns of the Simple, Complex, and Integrated Models are understood, they can be applied to even the subtlest of movements.

Chapter 10

The Challenges of Change

Change Is Big!

Since you are reading this book, you might be interested in finding information that can lead to some kind of change. We believe the Framework provides movers of all abilities, ages, and cultural backgrounds with an adaptive structure and tools that help identify habits and encourage a more *sentient, patterned, and choice-based* approach to change in daily activities as well as specialized movement. We hope that as you have progressed through these chapters, questions have arisen and you have had sparks of awareness and insight about yourself and others. We hope you have playfully and lightly approached some movement explorations, interacted with some of the suggested props, and watched videos and interviews that support your inquiries and curiosity. Have you experienced a change in your awareness of your body, a way of thinking, or an actual physical difference while working with Framework for Integration?

Change is Fundamental—The essence of movement is change. But this change is not random. In the process of development, change is both relational and patterned. You can change your current movement patterns by revisiting early patterns. And, since it is axiomatic that change is inevitable, you will change, whether you want to or not. The question then becomes how much you want to actively choose in which ways you will change or in which ways you will interact with the change.

—Peggy Hackney, *Making Connections: Total Body Integration Through Bartenieff Fundamentals*

Change is a mammoth and universal topic! It can't be denied; it is all around us—in our bodies, our environment, our shifting life circumstances, and accompanying emotions. But knowing something is inevitable or logical doesn't always make it easy to experience. There are so many different facets of change. Sometimes, if and when we see a need for it, we embrace it, want it. Sometimes a partner, parent, teacher, physician, or coach tells us we need to change—our lives and well-being may depend on smaller, cumulative changes or maybe a big, drastic one. Consumer capitalism would have no fuel or sway if it didn't exploit our doubts about changing ourselves. We subscribe often to the stories that tell us that if we change our diets, possessions, fashion, way of life, location, or job, we might finally grasp that elusive peace, satisfaction, power, or love we crave. In the face of inescapable change, say, watching our children grow up, experiencing our aging, or coming to terms with death and loss, we often resist or become numb to it. Sometimes we don't think we can muster the requisite inspiration and energy to change, and sometimes the process of change is so subtle and stealthy that we find ourselves changed without being able to directly trace how it happened.

Joan Murray liked to tell the story of how initially resistant she was to the Alexander Technique. Feeling dragged along to lessons by her husband, Alex, after some time, she recalled a vivid moment of looking in a mirror and not recognizing the person looking back—she was so changed. She often repeated a saying credited to the famous Buddhist priest, philosopher, and poet Dōgen: "When you walk in the mist, you get wet." Change is like that. Walking through the mist of our lives, we too might recognize that we have learned and changed a lot without directly tracking how or when. We might also tell stories of a time or two when all the right elements converged at the right moment in the right context and BOOM, the change we experienced was nearly instantaneous.

From the Framework's developmental perspective, whether ontogenetic or phylogenetic, a consistent thread throughout is that though there may be exceptions, generally, *change takes time*—in the case of evolution and adaptation, sometimes eons. Insight and recognition may happen in a flash of understanding, but the time it takes to undo, unlearn, learn, and rewire the brain's proverbial hard drive and accompanying cultural "software" might take longer than liked or planned. Anyone who has ever rehabbed from a serious bodily injury, exited an untenable living environment, or grieved a deep loss has experienced this; modification to the new normal, healing, and progress are hard-won and take patient commitment.

Somatic Learning Environment

The Framework's many interlacing elements come from a mix of anthropological, therapeutic, and somatic sources that hold space for gradual but powerful change. The Laban/Bartenieff, Alexander Technique, and developmental movement foundations all emphasize what physical therapist and renowned somatic educator Glenna Batson calls "a somatic learning environment" that reflects certain perspectives on time, mindfulness, and non-judgment (2009, 4). Slowing down helps us to reflect on the layers of detail in even the simplest movement experience: "Somatic approaches emphasize sensory awareness (paying attention to sensing) over motor action ('doing'). In the somatic learning context, how one moves is more important than what the movement is" (Batson 2009, 4). This simple definition is counter to our results-based culture that often demands, from a misinformed vantage point, that *change should manifest immediately and at any cost.* In the reality of motor learning and learning in general, having time to reflect and rest gives "the nervous system time for processing and integration and physiological systems time to recover" (Batson 2009, 5). Time to experience, time to reflect, time to rest after acting, and time to integrate information are key to lasting change.

Consciousness and Habit

In his book *Subliminal: How Your Unconscious Mind Rules Your Behavior,* theoretical physicist Leonard Mlodinow says, "It can be difficult to distinguish willed, conscious behavior from that which is habitual or automatic" (2012, 12) and asserts that most human beings are overly confident about their level of conscious awareness, as well as their ability to make fully independent and conscious choices. He documents studies during which people insisted they were consciously remembering, choosing, or discerning when they absolutely were not. Even worse, in one controlled experiment, participants were asked to share their remembrances of the order of events and actions as they happened. When presented with video evidence that their actions and choices were not actually how they remembered them, rather than questioning their perceptions, some angrily questioned the veracity of the experiment's video record! This anecdote relates directly to the Alexander Technique principle of Unreliable Sensory Appreciation; in human beings, unconscious suggestion and habits are far stronger drivers than conscious choice.

As previously discussed, another hallmark of the Alexander Technique is its attention to and respect for the power of habit. Though often framed negatively, habits are brilliant mechanisms that automate simple and repeated motor tasks in efficiently distributed areas of the central nervous system so the frontal cortex doesn't have to over-expend energy learning and relearning. The grooves of habit are a double-edged sword. On one hand, habits (automation) free up our brains to engage in complex thinking that includes, among many possibilities, assessing contexts, making meaning, creative imagination, critical thinking, and problem-solving. On the other hand, deeply ingrained habits often hijack our best intentions when we want or need to change. As Mlodinow asserts, the rub is when we think we are consciously making choices and decisions when we actually aren't. Or, from an Alexander Technique perspective, this is when we consciously want or decide to change, but unconscious habits of body and mind derail our attempts.

To change, we have to come to terms with the idea that our habits manifest in lifelong *patterns* that have their roots in numerous internal and external relationships. Author Peggy Hackney suggests that though we enter the world as unified beings, acclimating to the environments into which we are born begins with the process of differentiating our parts—a necessary developmental process that eventually leads to integrating an understanding of our whole self (2002, 11).

It takes an infant some time to realize that the small hand waving back and forth in front of her face is actually *her* hand; through varied experiences, successes, and failures, she learns, "Oh, this is *my* hand." Then, in her journey toward integration, responding and relating back and forth between her internal sensations and her external environment, she relates that knowledge back to the whole: "My hand is part of *me*." She will adapt to the version of the world she's been brought into; her culture, race, abilities, gender, class, opportunities, and traumas will dictate how her habits of thought and movement crystallize. If she has the ability and opportunity to learn to speak and read, her earlier embodied, nonverbal awareness will be sublimated to the task of language acquisition (Moore and Yamamoto 1988, 85). After late childhood, the way she experiences and thinks about the world will be conspicuous in how she moves her body (or doesn't). Her health and functionality throughout the lifespan, as well as how she ages, will reflect all the development (or lack of development) that has gone before. And the bulk of all these processes will have been laid down at a largely unconscious level.

Interferences with Change

The realm of the habitual unconscious is probably the foremost disruptor of our capacity to change. Experiencing enormously difficult life challenges, especially in childhood (adverse childhood experiences or "ACEs"[1]), can lead to the body and mind carrying deep and ongoing effects of suffering that stay sublimated and wreak havoc on our health and overall well-being. In the aftermath of the COVID-19 pandemic, we can no longer deny this specter of trauma, if we were inclined to before. This book is not about trauma—many brilliant researchers and healers are writing about the topic.[2] It is mentioned here briefly because sustaining the characteristics of authentic, lasting learning depends so closely on environments that support optimal equilibrium of the nervous system. Learning is the catalyst for change, reflected in observable aspects of curiosity, emotional connection, and personal relevance (Lahey 2016).

For a clear picture of what trauma is (and isn't), in his book *My Grandmother's Hands: Racialized Trauma and the Pathway to Mending Our Hearts and Bodies*, Resmaa Menakem guides:

> Trauma always happens in the body. It is a spontaneous protective mechanism used by the body to stop or thwart further (or future) potential damage.

> . . . It is a highly effective tool of safety and survival. Trauma is also not an event. Trauma is the body's protective response to an event—or a series of events—that it perceives as potentially dangerous. This perception may be accurate, inaccurate, or entirely imaginary. . . . An embedded trauma response can manifest as fight, flee, or freeze—or as some combination of constriction, pain, fear, dread, anxiety, unpleasant (and/or sometimes pleasant) thoughts, reactive behaviors, or other sensations or experiences. . . . We can have a trauma response to anything we perceive as a threat, not only to our physical safety, but to what we do, say, think, care about, believe in or yearn for . . . trauma is also a wordless story our body tells itself about what is safe and what is a threat (2017, 8).

Often, in somatic learning, in our earnest desire to practice something new or change, when we slow down the pace and explore unfamiliar movement experiences and patterns, if we have the "stuck" energy of trauma in our bodies, we may experience unfamiliar emotional and physical occurrences. We might feel minor irritation, frustration, or fatigue. Other times, waves of intense emotions—deep grief, overwhelming fear, or rage—might surface and be experienced alongside shaking, trembling, shivering, muscular tension, weakness, or pain (Levine and Frederick 1997, 38, 58, 97–98; Levine 2010, 4–9). Modernity posits that the body is a mechanized conglomeration of fixable and replaceable parts that can be transplanted to any environment undisrupted. But we don't experience our lives that way. When we travel or experience a substantive life shift, we are surprised by our fatigue and the time it takes to adjust; we often think, "What is wrong with me? Why do I feel so tired, sluggish, strange, emotional, etc.?" For those who have encountered debilitating stress and trauma, change may take more time and trust.

If, with some of the movement explorations in the Simple, Complex, or Integrated Models, there have been experiences of even momentary disruption in senses of safety or equilibrium, it might be time to pay close attention to the messages the body/mind is sending. Working on the physioball might disrupt or unsettle a sense of balance. As the body struggles to remap the location and actions of the pelvis, this crucial and sensitive part of the body can send a lot of signals. Locked hip joints, overly stretched or tight spinal muscles, spasmed pelvic floors, and generalized tension abound in twenty-first-century bodies. Movement here might feel unfamiliar, restricted, or dangerous, especially balancing on a mobile platform. The Framework provides enough structure for the mover to take calculated risks inside a general sense of orientation and safety. Because most people have already experienced developmental movement in infancy, toddlerhood, and early childhood—albeit without the purposeful consciousness now possible—this movement reiterates a sense of familiarity, even in less flexible or adaptable adult bodies.

> **The psychology of the adult human being is an unfolding, ever-emergent process marked by subordination of older behavior systems to new, higher order systems. . . . Each successive stage or level of existence is a state through which people may pass on the way to other states of equilibrium.**
>
> **—Dr. Clare Graves, *The Never Ending Quest***

Stages of Change

In applying Framework for Integration toward goals of change, it seems important to reiterate that "behavioral change is often nonlinear; progression and regression are common in stages of change" (Silver and Worthington 2021). The willingness to change and the states of mind that change depends on have been outlined in various psychosocial models. The stages of change we have seen active in our journeys in dance, becoming Alexander Technique teachers, recovering from injuries, and many other contexts often have been in this order, adapted from the Transtheoretical Model:

- The dawning of awareness or concern about wanting or needing to change.
- The growing awareness crystallizing into a commitment or intention to change.
- Commitment and intention leading to the continued curiosity, exploration, and action that supports change.
- Like Joan, experiencing the realization that after some time in a supported structure or community, habits of thinking and body have changed.
- Maintaining awareness, patience, and self-forgiveness during frustrating plateaus and regressions when the changes seem lost or unclear.

People can interrupt their habits, and with the help of clear structures, create new patterns that support their desires for integrated health and wholeness. As we have incorporated the Framework into our own lives and teaching, we have found that the Simple, Complex, and Integrated Models are everywhere we look, whether in simple, daily moments like brushing our teeth or teaching dance students a complex coordination or phrase of choreography. Learning something transformative or paradigm shifting makes it impossible to return to "not knowing"—everything has changed.

Change can be exciting, exhilarating, joyful, and empowering! In a world where so much of what is decided and happens is out of one's control, finding the ability to consciously direct the current of change in body and mind is both adaptive and grounding. This is especially true when experiencing the effects of aging; more tools and conscious awareness are needed to live life to the fullest. We offer the Framework as a clear structure that supports the desire for change.

With hope and encouragement, we offer this recapitulation and pose some questions to consider:

1. For the rest of your life, learning and change are inevitable! Welcome!
2. Somatic learning leads to powerful and lasting change by asking you to slow down, tune in, and refrain from judgment.
    - Do you have unreasonable expectations for your capacity to change (and where did these originate)?
    - If lasting movement change is important to you, how might you prioritize finding some time for a somatic learning process?
3. Habits just are—don't make them your enemy. Rather, hold a healthy respect for their efficiency and power while also practicing a more conscious awareness of them.
    - How are you moving from unconscious movement habit to clearer conscious awareness?
    - How might your movement relate to the ways you generally see the world?
    - What is working for you?
    - What is no longer working for you?
    - As you observe yourself, does self-condemnation or high internal pressure keep showing up?
4. Throughout our lives, we keep differentiating our many parts and relating them back to the greater whole of ourselves. The parts can include many things, for example, actual body parts and systems, our emotions, and our varying states of mind.
    - What are the ways you see your parts and whole?
    - How is your self-concept or identity influenced by your culture, race, gender, ability, or age?
    - Are there aspects of your self-definition and identity that are no longer useful or supportive, or are getting in the way of the change you desire?
    - Where can you find practices and communities that support the changes you want to make?
5. Trauma's residue in the body/mind can interfere with meaningful, engaged physical learning when the structure or environment doesn't feel safe and activates fight, flight, freeze, and other responses.
    - When you enter a new learning environment, is your initial experience fearful?
    - Do fear and/or anxiety make you resistant to change?

- Might previous traumatic experiences be a possible source of that resistance?
- If so, how might you move forward with addressing it?
- What communities and resources can support you?
- As you become aware of the ways you want to experience change, remember that all change takes time, is progressive but non-linear, encompasses many stages, including regression, but can also be transformative and empowering!
- How might you extend patience toward yourself as you experience varying levels of awareness, intention, decision-making, action, and seeming backward motion? (If you find yourself unable to act, circle back to No. 4.)

NOTES

1. For more information on adverse childhood experiences, see Harvard University's Center on the Developing Child article "ACEs and Toxic Stress: Frequently Asked Questions": https://developingchild.harvard.edu/resources/aces-and-toxic-stress-frequently-asked-questions/. A great website that gives more history and cites ongoing studies about the statistical relationships between ACEs and adult depression, addiction, chronic pain, and more is here: https://acestoohigh.com/got-your-ace-score/.
2. Authors writing about trauma: Bessel van der Kolk, Resmaa Menakem, Staci K. Haines, Peter Levine, Daniel Siegel, Dr. Stephen Porges, among many others.

Chapter 11
Breathing

> **Breath is the bridge which connects life to consciousness, which unites your body to your thoughts.**
>
> **—Thich Nhat Hanh, *The Miracle of Mindfulness: An Introduction to the Practice of Meditation***

Breathing is an omnipresent part of our everyday movement and, as such, is an integral part of any activity we undertake. In popular movement practices as well as specialized professional work, we often are asked to breathe on cue to address perceived holding and muscular tension, build technical prowess, and relieve shortness of breath or anxiety. Breathing often is treated as a localized function—we pay focused attention to the diaphragm, belly, ribs, lungs, and the trunk in general. Framework for Integration investigates where habits interfere with efficient functioning throughout the whole body, though this approach is not prescriptive.

Many ideas exist about the use of breath in speech and vocal training, wind instrument pedagogies, and yoga practices. The Framework viewpoint is not disputing varied approaches to breathing but rather offering an entrance into a way to connect breath to *use*—an Alexander Technique/developmental perspective. This chapter opens the door to explore different possibilities around habitual ways of breathing and offers ways to rethink and reclaim breath.

Breathing is a rather simply defined process. There are miles of air pressure above our heads; to breathe in, we only need to allow the air to come into the thoracic cavity. Yet, if breathing is brought to our awareness, many of us get overly self-conscious and automatically interfere with these simple physics. Anxiety around paying attention to breathing is common. In a variety of contexts, we often are asked to demonstrate that we are breathing, whether being asked to "take a deep breath" at the doctor's office or the prescribed breath in a yoga or Pilates class. Many current practices have us habitually inhale in a Secondary orientation. This encourages forcing or sucking air into the lungs while arching our spines and distending our ribs. Other systems believe in holding the breath to gain a certain amount of stored or momentary power. Breath is the mirror of overall use intended to support the needed level of activity.

Much common thought around breathing views it as a local event situated in the abdomen or ribs but rarely shared throughout the whole. In the Framework, breathing is meant to be experienced throughout the whole body. If, for example, we put hands on an ankle and can't sense the subtle changes breath is affecting, the breath might be meeting some interference and not reverberating throughout.

Alexander: "The Breathing Man"

F. M. Alexander worked on removing interferences to breathing and was known as the "Breathing Man" early in his career. He designed a procedure called the "Whispered Ah" which helped organize the student to notice any extra muscular work while exhaling an "Ah" sound. The process asks the student to juggle attention during the exhale—adding a subtle smile while placing the tip of the tongue on the lower teeth. The teacher monitors the exhale, watching to see if the student can sustain the overall length of the torso as the ribs soften and narrow and then expand, bouncing back to invite the inhale.

In the "Whispered Ah," the exhale is an Engagement followed by a Reset. A Reset inhale encourages air to flow in with little effort. In terms of Engagements and Resets, breath can of course be more complex. At the Simple Model level, the general lengthening associated with exhaling can be seen as a Secondary. At the Complex level, the whole web of spirals condenses to produce a narrowing of the trunk's musculature to expel the air, after which air easily flows back in during a Reset. At the Integrated level, the exhale becomes a Secondary Ball Forward (*Seagulls*) as air goes out and a Secondary Ball Back (*Ocean*) as air rushes back in. In considering the antagonistic action of the Upper and Lower Triangles, engaging or grounding the Lower Triangle in an exhale (abdominals and pelvic floor up through the head) frees the Upper Triangle (including the diaphragm), which then readies itself to reengage, in turn supporting the Lower Triangle in a Reset and creating the vacuum that allows air to refill the lungs. Each of these models will be explored in the movement explorations below.

Since breathing is so habitually ingrained, so sensitive in nature, and so unconscious in daily activity, it is important to not be heavy handed in considering interferences. The lighter the approach, the better. Directing your thinking is truly your best friend in approaching breath. If looking at breath from any of the models feels too complicated and/or brings about anxiety, the best approach is to let it go. We support working/practicing in a responsible, non-demanding manner that honors Alexander's principle of Inhibition.

In the following movement explorations, remember that the body's orientation of "up," *ball* forward, *ball* back, and others have changed in space. In supine, prone, or on all fours, spatially reorienting to the body as the map (such as top of head, feet, and front body) will clarify Primary and Secondary intents.

Whole Body Breathing: Supine, Prone, and on All Fours

MOVEMENT EXPLORATION 11.1:
BREATHING IN CONSTRUCTIVE REST (SUPINE)

Lie on your back with a book under your head, your knees bent, and your hands on your abdomen. Get comfortable with your own breathing, track it for a while, and begin to see if any patterns of the Simple Model in Primary and Secondary become noticeable. Does turning your attention to your breath invoke any surprising or unwelcome states of mind? (For example: "This is very relaxing, I love doing this!" or "Paying attention to this is making me anxious.") Do you have ideas about the inhale or the exhale or of what "should" happen during either? Mentally bookmark those ideas. Are you noticing habits? (For example, are your respirations even, faster, slower, or uneven?) Do you prefer one phase of a breath over the other?

Without judgment, being familiar with your own breath patterning and habits is really important. Are you noticing any clear Primary or Secondary? Now let's turn our attention to the Framework models:

1. Simple Model: Encourage a general Primary as you inhale. Send your attention to your back ribs and your thoracic and sacral spinal curves (mid and lower back). This is very different from cultural ideas of paying attention to the front ribs lifting up. Your back may seem more pronounced, rounding into the surface on which you are lying. Release your head while gently grounding your heels.

2. Complex Model: As you attend to your inhale and exhale, imagine the double helix muscular structure opening and closing in waves. Lying on the floor encourages the thoracic to extend and lengthen during the *exhale*, while the *inhale* encourages the lumbar to open up three-dimensionally.

3. Integrated Model: Try the exhale as a Secondary Ball Forward (*Seagulls*) and the inhale as a Secondary Ball Back (*Ocean*). Remember that because your orientation in space has changed, looking "up" will be looking along the ceiling and then almost behind you. During the exhale, your legs can gently push from your feet to propel the pelvis up through the spine to the head as the pelvis releases slightly forward, as if the *ball* were rolling forward (no more than a thought). Here, the Upper Triangle Resets, freeing the arms and upper body as the Lower Engages to support the weight of the pelvis and legs. In the inhale, the Lower Triangle will Reset, the legs will free, and the Upper Triangle will stabilize.

MOVEMENT EXPLORATION 11.2: BREATHING PRONE

Have one or two pillows available that you can place under your chest and hips as you lie on the floor (optional if they prove uncomfortable). You also might want to have a book or rolled-up towel on which you can place your forehead, high enough so that your nose doesn't press into the floor. Place your forehead on the ground, towel, or book, tuck your wrists in the crease of your hips, elbows bent, with your legs inwardly rotated, heels falling out. Notice your comfort or lack of comfort. As in Movement Exploration 4.1, this position generally emphasizes all the Primary contours of the body: head, front of shoulders, elbows, back of wrists, and knees contacting the ground and finally, the tops of the feet as they supinate. After a while, let yourself include the breath in your awareness. Where are you feeling the breath? Do you notice an increase in Primary or Secondary? Anywhere in particular in your body? Are you feeling your ribs moving? Are you feeling your lower back/abdomen push into the floor? Is your neck getting tense? Don't do too much about what you are observing.

Now align exhales with overall whole-body Secondary. This means that as you exhale, start *thinking* about looking up, and reinforce this thought with a slight pressure on the forearms that helps you lengthen the trunk and support the head/neck. At the same time, the legs will tend to externally rotate, powering overall length from the bottom of the pelvis through the spine. It will take a relaxed, prolonged exhale to line up all of this in one exhale. Once done, let go of all Secondary activity, even the wish to get it right, into a Reset that brings you into a refreshed Primary. Repeat the process a few times, always aiming at doing as little as possible—only the hint of a Secondary throughout the whole is necessary.

Next, shift your focus to align your inhale with overall whole-body Primary. This means that as you inhale, start *thinking* about looking down, and reinforce this thought with a slight pressure on the head and forearms that helps you curve the trunk and support the pelvis to leave the floor. At the same time, allow the legs to internally rotate, releasing the pelvis up and back from the floor, allowing the knees to bend and the whole body to respond. It will take a relaxed, prolonged inhale to line up all of this in one inhale. Once done, let go of all Primary activity into a Reset that brings you into a refreshed Secondary. Repeat the process a few times—only the hint of a Primary is necessary.

Once you feel comfortable with both halves of the movement exploration, try to link them together:

While exhaling, associate it with overall Secondary.

While inhaling, associate it with overall Primary.

MOVEMENT EXPLORATION 11.3: BREATHING ON ALL FOURS

Once you have thought this through on your back and prone, you can try it on all fours in all three models. The breathing should be reflected through the limbs and will also encourage a movement forward toward the head and back toward the hips, which is in direct relationship to Movement Explorations 8.2 and 8.4 (you are essentially layering breath into these exercises). As usual, it's up to you to pick which model works best for your understanding.

1. Simple Model: If, as we have been doing, we align exhale with Secondary and inhale with Primary, shifting weight to the upper limbs will be the exhale, and the inhale will shift weight toward the lower limbs.

2. Complex Model: The double-spiral musculature of the trunk three-dimensionally narrows on the exhale, as weight shifts to the upper limbs (with a "pull" in hands and wrists) and expands on the Resetting inhale as weight shifts to the lower limbs (more "push" in hands and wrists).

3. Integrated Model: In the exhale, the weight shifts to the upper limbs and the Upper Triangle Engages, grounding the upper torso and freeing the lower limbs and pelvis (can you wiggle your legs a little?). The *ball* is in Secondary Ball Forward (*Seagulls*). In the Reset inhale, the weight shifts to the lower limbs and the Lower Triangle Engages, grounding the pelvis and legs and freeing up the arms and shoulder girdle (can you wiggle your arms/elbows a little?). The *ball* is in Secondary Ball Back (*Ocean*).

On all fours, maintaining an awareness of supporting the head and pelvis "up and back" is always helpful. As you fatigue, it is easy for the head to droop below the line of your clavicles (face to the floor) and the lower back to collapse into an over-accentuated arch. Both of these habits will interfere with efficient breath patterning.

If you have found these three breathing explorations revealing of your ways of thinking about breath as well as your habits, stay with them. Any time spent resting in supine or prone can be directed to the action of breathing without having to stay with it for too long. If you have enjoyed exploring breath in supine, prone, and on all fours, and you are ready to juggle multiple layers of attention as well as your balance, you can try aligning these patterns with the Four Phases on the ball.

Integrated Model: Four Phases

MOVEMENT EXPLORATION 11.4: BREATHING PHASES ON THE BALL

In this movement exploration, we decide to continue relating the phases of breathing with phases of the ball work—Primary will be associated with inhaling and Secondary will be linked to exhaling. Begin by exhaling, then move through a–e.

a. In Primary Ball Forward (*Beach Chair*), inhale as the ball goes forward.
b. In Primary Ball Back (*Sandals*), continue to inhale as you switch the ball to go back.
c. In Secondary Ball Back (*Ocean*), Reset the breath into an exhale, with the ball continuing to go back.
d. In Secondary Ball Forward (*Seagulls*), continue the exhale with the ball now going forward.
e. Repeat and see if you can continue syncing the breath with moving the ball.

Feel free to stay in a phase longer with additional breaths if moving from phase to phase seems too rapid a process. Move to the next phase only when you feel comfortable.

Upper and Lower Triangles

The final movement exploration focuses solely on the Upper and Lower Triangle paradigm in the Integrated Model. Here we demonstrate how the breath can be associated with a cyclic Engagement and Reset of the triangles as well as alternately freeing the upper and lower limbs. Though complex, we include the application for those who want to work further in this particular model.

MOVEMENT EXPLORATION 11.5:
UPPER AND LOWER TRIANGLES IN BREATHING

Lie on your back, arms above your shoulders, with legs bent, feet on the floor. Imagine your hands are holding onto a pull-up bar above your head. We are aiming for a general open Secondary pattern in the upper and a Primary pattern in the lower. Quietly allow the breath to stabilize while paying attention to the Upper and Lower Triangles. During an exhale, slowly and gently start to bend your elbows. As you bend your elbows, allow the spine to subtly lengthen toward the imaginary bar. Take care to *not* "anchor" or pull the shoulder blades down toward the hips—the sensation of your elbows bending is key and supersedes any action of the shoulders. The gentle pull to the elbows will create an Engagement of the Upper Triangle. To encourage the lengthened Secondary here, as you pull to the elbows, you can also think of looking up to the space between your eyebrows. You may feel your torso traveling up toward your head. In coordination with the end of the exhale, at the end of the pull, allow the inhale to Reset that action as the weight transfers back to the lower body—this release may feel like a rocking back toward your feet. As the inhale's Engagement phase gets under way, notice the support and weight of the legs and pelvis. As the exhale begins again, the action of bending the elbows will start the cycle again, Engaging the Upper Triangle to Reset the Lower. Continue to pay attention to the exchange of upper and lower action until the antagonistic relationship between Upper and Lower Triangles becomes more and more apparent: when one is Engaging, the other is Resetting. Notice that the two overlap—one doesn't finish completely before the other starts.

Summary

We offered this work in Part Four: Synthesis because it contains a complex integration of the Framework's concepts overall. This is the Framework's application at its most subtle: breathing as a movement microcosm of Framework layered lenses and the preceding movement explorations. In working with breathing, throughout this chapter, we decided to assign certain affinities with certain actions, but it is not prescriptive. In all the explorations above, no matter the lens, *either an exhale or an inhale can start as an Engagement and finish as a Reset.* The Framework approach may take some time practicing with these concepts to become comfortable.

We trust our approach aligns with many breathing practices, from yogic *pranayama,* to voice work, to Alexander's focus on breath, to the most recent neuroscientific and psychotherapeutic breathing techniques that address stress and trauma and encourage a parasympathetic response or calming of the nervous system. We assert that the exercises in prone with the emphasis on Primary patterning particularly encourage rest and Resetting. We hope this work will help you identify habits that may be preventing you from enjoying the full range of breath that is your birthright.

Chapter 12

Wrap-Up

Throughout its development, Framework for Integration has been an ongoing process of synthesizing "diverse conceptions into a coherent whole" and will continue to be long after this book is published. Circling back to Ken Wilber's ideas about ongoing development, the Framework endeavors to reflect how a coherent but flexible whole can help support all sorts of people and their goals for ongoing change.

Synthesis: the combining of often diverse conceptions into a coherent whole; the dialectic combination of thesis and antithesis into a higher stage of truth.

—www.merriam-webster.com

Change starts precisely where one finds oneself in any given moment. It is not a future event; it is now. Each breath has its own rhythm, pattern, and purpose and is an opportunity to be in the now, paying attention. Every moment of our lives is in developmental flux. Through the din of the many voices vying for our attention, ultimately, we must become the experts of our own lives and bodies. Developmental processes and aging are happening whether we pay attention or not.

If we approach our goals and desire for change without a sense of Alexandrian Inhibition, we might forget that we ourselves are a coherent whole and not merely an assemblage of relative parts. Without patience and pause, we have the propensity to laser-focus our creativity and adaptability in ways that can potentially hurt us and ultimately aren't sustainable. By putting aside right and wrong binaries and observing ourselves patiently, we can build practices of inhibition and direction (and redirection) so that we can more skillfully assess the appropriate approach for our immediate circumstances.

Once we recognize and accept the responsibility of being in charge of our own relationship to awareness and development, it is important to assess whether:

1. What we are doing is what we *intended* to do.
2. *Without judgment*, we are allowing for modifications grounded in our observations.
3. We are allowing for the process to be flexible and ongoing, without too much force of effort.

The crux of *synthesis* is that when it happens, the integration of information is so deep and thorough that former thinking and organization must give way to an entirely revised or new structure. This is learning. Persisting and staying present with ourselves in this deconstruction-to-reconstruction paradigm engenders deepening trust and confidence in our capacity to effect lasting change in multiple spheres. Working with our breathing or considering how we are approaching the rhythmic phrasing of our movement tasks are opportunities to observe integration and synthesis in real time. On the waves of the sea of change, we all pulse with the shifting tides, anticipating the right moment to stand and surf. Being more conscious of how we are using and experiencing our whole selves builds the sensitivity and trust necessary to ride the waves of life's changes into healthier, more adaptive movement choices. This is the Framework's purpose and path.

Part Five

Applications

Introduction

Sprinkled throughout the previous chapters are quotes, anecdotes, and observations from others whose experiences working with Framework for Integration have illuminated or changed their understanding of their movement practice habits and choices. With those stories as prelude, we like to think of Part Five as getting down to the bedrock and purpose of Framework for Integration: its real-time, real-world application across a range of everyday tasks as well as specialized professional practices.

In Chapter Thirteen, building on his experience with researching wheelchair design efficacy, Luc shares more of his thoughts about the impact that design has on human movement overall. While modern designs and technologies intend to keep us safer, might they also be interfering with how we naturally learn and build physical skills?

Chapter Fourteen looks at Framework applications and lenses across a wide variety of everyday tasks, activities, and recreational sports. From walking to driving, gardening to chopping wood, the Framework models can help direct choice, mindful efficiency, and ease. We, the authors, delight in exploring the models in our recreative and recuperative moments as we kayak, ride bicycles, or work out in a group fitness class. Though the possibilities are endless, we have included ample examples, which we hope readers will apply and proverbially (and literally!) "run with," finding additional ways to apply Framework thinking to an ever-expanding range of activities.

Chapters Fifteen to Eighteen gather together essays from contributors applying Framework for Integration across a range of professions and backgrounds, featuring in their own words how they use the concepts and practices. We are thrilled to share their thoughts and exciting work, as well as some of our own specific practices in mindfulness meditation, fitness class, and yoga. Most of our collaborators in these chapters are also Alexander Technique teachers; we look forward to publishing future work that addresses how the Framework specifically informs AT pedagogy and teacher training.

Friends and colleagues on three continents have shared in the formation and language of this work. Some saw immediate applications after one workshop; most are what we call "lifers" committed to growing the work daily (see Acknowledgments). We are so grateful for their trust, support, and ultimately, the faith in the way the system reconnects us all to our ancestry as mammals and human beings. Together, we honor and share in the legacy of many of our somatic ancestors and influences. So much of the work Rudolf Laban is credited with was actually explored and articulated by his closest students, the evolution of F. M. Alexander's work was carried forward by many in his inner circle, and so it goes in our own experience.

Longtime student and colleague of Joan and Alex Murray, Rebecca, teaches Luc and Elizabeth, who then share through their own teaching. Our students become our collaborators (and coauthors!) and, of course, even our own teachers. In the spirit of the Murrays paraphrased, "You are just getting ready to learn," and more important, "You will make this your own." We hope that as you explore the Framework in your daily life and activities, you will discover something new, make it your own, and share it with others.

Chapter 13

The Impact of Design on Movement Skill

> **Intelligence: a person or being with the ability to acquire and *apply* knowledge.**
>
> **—Oxford Languages**

This chapter explores our reciprocal relationship with design, where the motivation to make our lives easier can lessen our capacity to be responsive and alert. For example, we design smooth sidewalks so that we can all walk more safely outside our homes, and yet, the even surfaces also dull our senses as we walk, so that we may be likely to trip and fall if even one small area is uneven. In our daily movement interactions with buildings, computers, cars, tools, and people, our bodies get taught to respond habitually. A cellphone or a computer trains us to pay attention by sending us notifications. It's the same with online map programs, where someone might blindly follow the program's notifications rather than using it as a reference while staying aware of their surroundings. Social media constantly monitors our "likes" and adapts to our behaviors, tempting us to respond positively to more posts.

Alternately, video games guide us to be successful in various skills without actually having to use our body's movement, or by using movements that have little to do with success outside the video game world. And even more pernicious are designs that are meant to keep us safe, such as in cars, where new sensing technologies stop us from skidding while braking, no matter how hard we push on the brake pedal. We respond to warnings that we need to "steer" the car, when in fact, the technology can't accurately feel our hand pressure on the wheel, or we are warned to take a break when we are not driving in a way the car computer believes is "alert." While using these features is sensible, it also stops us from expanding our sensory feeling in relation to the car and its functions. We shape our technologies and they shape us right back, without us even realizing it. Just try driving a car without all the safety features that you have gotten used to and see how you feel. It can be disorienting and nerve wracking.

As described in the Introduction to Part Three, another example is the design of wheelchairs that demands the rider be banked in Primary for their safety, rather than giving them the possibility to respond to the push and pull needed to move the chair. Or the wheel and seat designs prioritize keeping the person in the chair "safe" rather than being responsive to their level of injury. These design flaws call for the person to adapt to a chair that is only occasionally serving their movement needs.

Other examples include household items from refrigerators to toothbrushes. Your continuous positive airway pressure (CPAP) machine is connected to the internet that tells your doctor how you are sleeping and how many hours you are using the machine. It can be connected to your phone, which also keeps track of your steps, blood pressure, and heart rate. How does that surveillance make you feel? And now, an electric toothbrush can easily give you feedback on whether you are applying too much pressure or not brushing long enough. This might be helpful if we all had the same bodies and habits, but since we don't, the technology may be discouraging us from developing a healthy attention to our own movement practices for the sake of safety, economics, or aesthetics. Rarely are we encouraged in these interactions to develop better skills, as we find ourselves reacting rather than responding.

To illustrate this, try to imagine a world where no matter what you did in terms of movement, some mechanism would step in and keep you safe. This would be like playing tennis with a ball that could never go outside the lines or hitting a nail with a hammer that could never miss. Skill would become somewhat useless, causing you to lose any sense of calibration. Attention would dull, and our overall "ability to acquire and apply knowledge and skills" would slowly disappear. Our intelligence would diminish, according to the Oxford Languages definition quoted above.

We are not independent agents separate from our environments. Our environments pose problems for us, stimulating our brains to become movement problem solvers. Our aptitude for moving needs a design that matches the interactivity between the environment and us. Sailing and canoeing, with their discriminating balance demands, are types of activities that call for our whole being to respond, accumulating knowledge and skill refinement with each repetition. This involves paying attention while aiming for specific results. But we currently find ourselves in a dilemma when it comes to this type of skill-building, now that our environments and tools are constantly being redesigned. Once we are no longer able to ascertain whether what we are doing is actually what we think we are doing, our ability to build skill becomes compromised. This is what happens when we play video games where we use our fingers to control whole characters and/or whole worlds. This is similar to surgeons who sit behind a machine, contorting their fingers to control automated functions to operate on sensitive body parts, either in the next room or across the globe on a battlefield. Such high-stress situations can interfere with breathing and encourage excess tension in the limbs for long periods of time, and yet, you can still be successful at the task (game or surgeries), only to find out later that your body is paying a high price.

In contrast, consider the beauty of tools created by tradespeople. These tools, designed in relationship to the living body, often have a different feel than mass-produced objects designed with cost, safety, or attractiveness alone in mind. Often, years of trial and error have gone into such designs, a living history of skill passed from master to apprentice. And as a result, we get an object in exquisite balance with the body, such as a Samurai sword, a piece of Shaker furniture, or a pair of First Nation moccasins—these designs reminding us that we are part of a greater whole. Even the field of ergonomics, with its research on the body's mechanics, often cannot produce products that match artisanal elegance in their use and form.

No matter what the design of the tool is, we want to understand how to engage with it in a way that allows us to see the optimal path to using the design. The tool might be deficient, but our response does not have to dull our senses. The real question becomes: Can we be smarter without physical skills? Without learning to calibrate our movements from day to day? We do not believe so. Design has the potential to help us grow from moment to moment. Ideally, design could be used to move us in a certain way to be successful and discourage us if we are not fully present and active—such as learning to use the well-balanced ax or risk hurting yourself. Only then can we continue to develop our relationship to attention and redirection within movement skill. This is not only about providing a desk with the proper height and knobs that appropriately fit our hands; it's about developing responsive designs that optimize opportunities for real-time feedback.

The reciprocal nature of design/technology and use of self prompts us to consider accountability and responsibility. The Framework is devised to support these kinds of inquiries. We may ask ourselves, "What does this design encourage in movement?" And then: "Is this an activity that would be facilitated by a push or a pull? Does my weight need to transfer to Engage or Reset? Where is the *ball* going? Does the design itself promote taking care of myself as I move within the activity? Does it support an exchange between using the Upper and Lower Triangles?" Imagine a world that would allow us to remain conscious and learning about ourselves as we went

So, no, AI won't blow up the world. But the increasingly uncritical embrace of it, in a variety of narrow contexts, means the gradual erosion of some of humans' most important skills.

—Nir Eisikovits, Professor of Philosophy and Director, Applied Ethics Center, UMass Boston

along. In this world, we would be able to take the time needed to handle a situation, redirect extra effort, and evaluate whether our original assumptions were useful. This is not a world where a sensor on your back keeps beeping to remind you to stand "straight" or where you turn to artificial intelligence to write your essays, but a world where regaining control of your movement skills allows you to reclaim poise and confidence in your overall being.

Chapter 14

Everyday Applications

First, a Word About Rest

Just as we attend to Engagements and Resets in the Framework, we also advocate for periods of work and periods of rest on a larger scale. That is, any movement practice could and should include attention to recuperation to counterbalance the work of physical activity. Rest allows the nervous system time for processing and integration (Batson 2009, 2). We suggest taking time each day to lie on your back, knees up and feet on the floor, with a book under your head, a position often referred to as Constructive Rest Position.[1] This position encourages the back to release to gravity, Resetting from habitual stresses and strains on the body. More specifically, it allows potentially excessive Secondary in the lower back and neck to rest, and potentially extra Primary in the upper back to lengthen. Once having recalibrated the body, you can consider approaching some of the activities you do on a daily basis. This can be exciting and rewarding, playfully bringing the mundane into consciousness, with the goal of mindfully working through these activities on your own, eventually reintegrating them back into your daily life.

For me, driving a car was always an enjoyable and playful activity.

—Guy Vanier, former Canadian Rally Racing Champion

All Models All the Time

All activities can be illustrated through all models. In this chapter, the order in which daily activities and recreational sports are discussed is determined by increasing complexity from Simple to Integrated Models. We hope to demonstrate

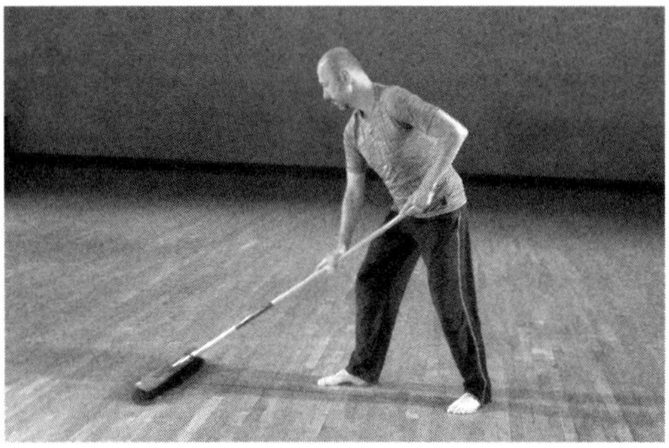

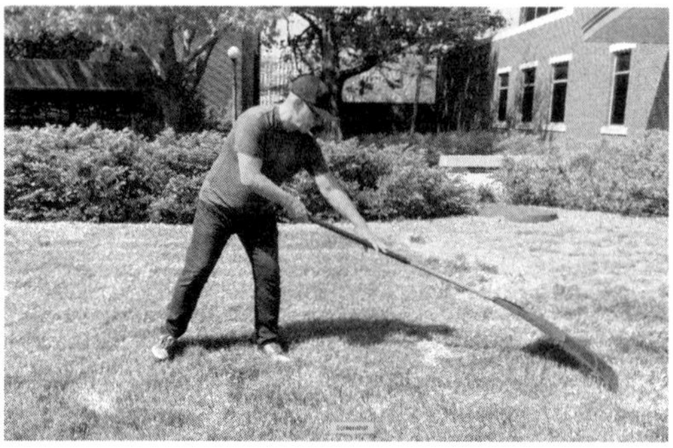

how one activity can be related to another inside of one model, with the possibility of revisiting it later through a different lens. Rather than analyzing each activity in each model, we relate and align similar activities with various models in an effort to empower the reader rather than provide dogmatic prescriptions.

Common tasks such as shoveling, stair climbing, walking, working on a computer, sweeping, raking, nailing, sawing, opening doors, climbing a ladder, driving a car, and turning a key can become enlivened when looked at from a new lens. In this section, the various models of the Framework are applied to many of these activities, from the everyday to sports and to physical training.

Video: Ladder Climbing

Paying Attention

Of all the various activities we do every day, inclining ourselves forward is perhaps one of the most common occurrences. Washing our hands, washing dishes, brushing our teeth, starting a bath, and leaning over a table, a patient, a counter, or the trunk of our car are all somewhat symmetrical actions, with the head inclined over the movement being carried out, looking either down or up, with the hip joints serving as counterweights. If you know your overall habitual tendencies in approaching this type of movement, you will be able to redirect yourself by asking whether you are in a Primary or Secondary. If you are inclined to be more toward Primary, looking up to lengthen in Secondary and then allowing an easy Reset will help undo the extra flexion over that sink. If your tendency is toward Secondary or trying to stay "straight," looking down and allowing a general softening might help rebalance the system. We can also transpose these movement strategies to typing on a computer, playing the piano, pushing a wheelbarrow, or leaning over a plate to eat. And, later, depending on your level of comfort with the Framework, you could switch models and start investigating the spirals or the ball work in all these activities. This will be explored further in the following examples in this chapter.

Asymmetrical tasks that we will consider include raking, shoveling, sweeping, nailing, sawing, opening doors, turning a key to unlock a door, weeding, and more. Here, the Complex Model is a good choice for observing your use in relation to what you have learned about the double spiral. It is useful to first be aware of your general tendencies—are you right or left handed? This will be a clue to your habitual patterns of favoring your dominant side. For example, in shoveling, notice which foot you step on to counterbalance the arms that are pushing the shovel into the dirt or the snow. That foot is meant to Engage in a Primary action. If you have the left foot forward, your right hand/arm will be in Primary and Engaging while plunging the shovel into the snow. Your left arm, while still on the shovel, will mainly be following the activity and Resetting, until you start to pull the shovel back and toss the snow over to one side or the other. Of course, shoveling can be done in many different ways.

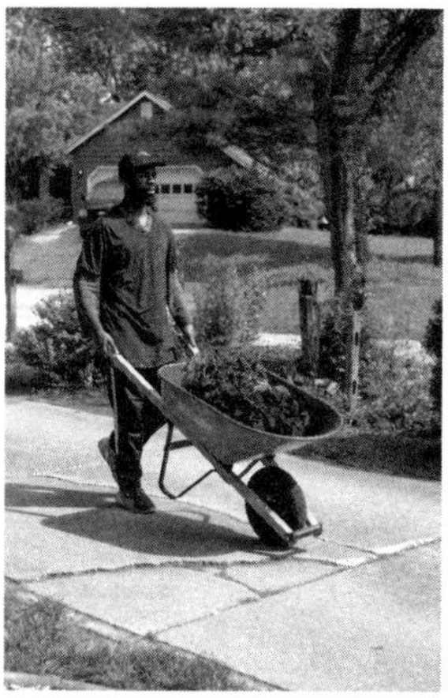

Symmetrical activity of pushing a wheelbarrow

The Integrated Model can also be applied to both of these examples—inclining over a sink and shoveling—but the Simple and Complex Models provide plenty to work with, and we encourage you to fully investigate those. It is also important to notice whether you are interfering with your breath during these activities, and if so, it might be helpful to notice where your weight is "parked," on either your legs or your arms. Take your time to get accustomed to your habitual way of handling the situation. There is no rush to change anything.

Gardening

Gardening is on the rise again, with cities setting up lots where residents can plant and harvest. Digging and raking topsoil, bending over to plant, weeding, and pulling vegetables out of the ground can be hard work. But the greater range of motion involved in working outside gives opportunities for noticing, evaluating, and possibly reorganizing your use inside these jobs. Remember to first revel in being outdoors, and don't rush through the tasks.

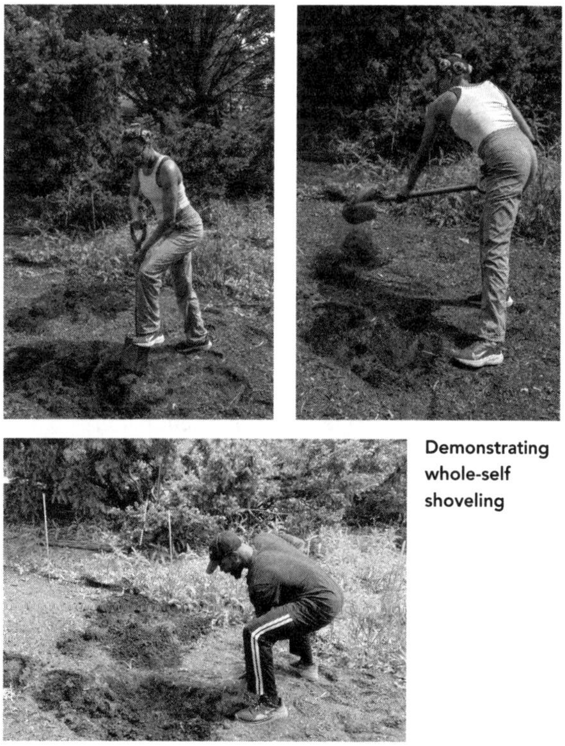

Demonstrating whole-self shoveling

Turning over the ground before planting can be relatively easy if you use your whole self with the shovel. Similar to the shoveling action described above, as you plant the shovel into the dirt, make sure that any force applied toward the ground is in Primary. If using your foot to push the shovel in, find the Primary Engagement of

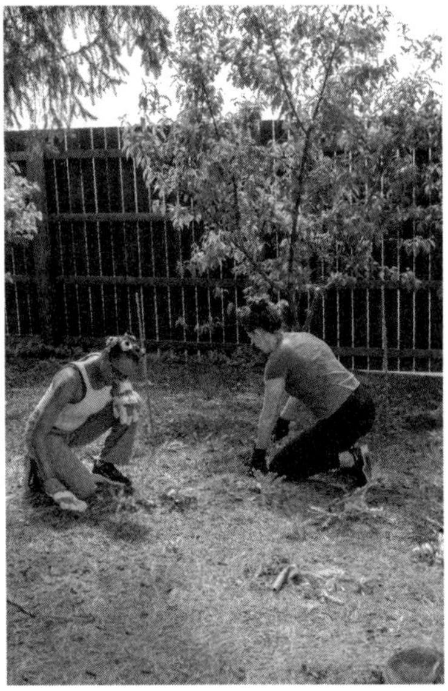

the heel and flexed foot as reflected all the way up through the spine. Then, pulling back the shovel is a Secondary activity, and tossing the dirt to the side is a Spiral. In doing jobs such as weeding or other tasks that require you to squat down to the ground, it is important that you release all extra Secondary work from the legs and lower back, because if you inadvertently hold on to Secondary in the lower body, your joints may feel tight and be difficult to bend. (It might be important to review Movement Exploration 8.5 about squatting before continuing.)

As the legs are bent in the squat, it is important to be able to push and pull with the arms with a supported upper back, usually in Secondary, in balance with the bend of the hip joints. As in Movement Exploration 8.5, where we explored squatting while pulling and pushing a chair, you might notice that in pushing a small trowel into the ground or pulling weeds, your upper back will alternate between Engagements and Resets. The Upper Triangle will necessarily be either Engaged or Reset in opposition to the Lower Triangle. Because squats can be especially challenging, we suggest using a low stool to help redirect the activity, or knee pads to facilitate putting a knee down on the ground. As you use your arms, keep their capacity to spiral in mind and notice, for example, if you are trying to pull a weed straight out of the ground versus spiraling it out. Try reaching out in pronation, grab the weed, and then pull it out in supination, allowing the elbow to bend while coming toward you. And as you pull, see if you can start the action at the hip, allowing the hip joint to provide a counterbalance to pull from. This is effectively about sending the *ball* back. In these extreme positions, it's important to notice whether the head is allowed to remain balanced and in opposition to the hips, providing the connective support to help pull the weed out of the ground. Gardening while thinking of your whole body is an art and makes it an event that keeps you healthy and grounded.

Driving

Driving a car is one of those activities where initially, one might not think it relates much to movement, and yet, once pointed out, it becomes impossible not to consider the movement patterns inherent in the seemingly simple act. Sitting in the driver's seat with both hands on the wheel encourages overall Primary. From an Integrated Model perspective, you would be in the *Beach Chair* phase with the *ball* going forward. The more you Engage with the wheel, the more the legs would tend to Reset. Pressing on either the gas or brake pedal will encourage movement of the *ball*. Since pressing on a pedal is an Engagement of the Lower, in theory, it would Reset the arms. Were you to pull yourself forward with your arms toward the windshield, your *ball* would be going back and your legs would Reset.

Driving is full of Spiraling activity, and any one-hand reach or pull in space will engender a spiral, requiring a transfer of weight, something that can be rather small and almost imperceptible but freeing, nevertheless. Turning right will require your right hand to pull the steering wheel while the left hand pushes it, usually alternating Engagements and Resets in the arms. Looking behind you to back up a car, swinging an arm around the passenger seat will trigger a weight transfer to either the right or left hip and facilitate a Secondary from one hip to shoulder and a Primary in the other. Notice if the arm that is swinging is pushing you into a spiral or pulling you into a spiral. This will directly affect the weight transfer (see Movement Exploration 5.2: Identifying Primary and Secondary in a Chair, Spiraling).

In the same way, pushing a pedal can happen in various ways, and it relates to the spiraling of the arms on the wheel. If sitting behind the wheel in *Beach Chair*, looking to accelerate while turning left, the extension of the right leg toward the pedal will create a Secondary from the right foot to the left shoulder, with your weight transferring to your left hip (with the *ball* escaping to the right with the centrifugal force). Explore on your own as to your preferred way to push a pedal while driving. As a side note, these explorations can be very useful to pianists who often spiral with the Upper Triangle while pushing a pedal with their right foot.

Finally, consider how you get in and out of the car. If people are being careful, normally they try to open the door and then symmetrically sit into the seat, and finally rotate to face the steering wheel. We suggest that getting into the car can be a spiral, as described in Movement Exploration 9.3 (Spirals in Transferring Weight While Standing). After opening the door to get in, think of taking the head away from the car, allowing the hips to lead into the seat, with the *ball* going away from the head. Getting out of the car is as in Movement Exploration 5.5 (Spiraling to Standing): As you open the door, allow the head to lead in a spiral and the body to follow. Taking a mindful approach to how you perform all these actions through the three models of the Framework can provide endless opportunities for refreshing your attention to this daily experience.

Video: Getting in and out of a Car with Spirals

Walking

Walking, as discussed in Movement Exploration 5.7, is a never-ending series of spirals, with the trunk continually switching from one spiral to another. Often, we see a diminished ability of the body to spiral when walking, and this has a negative impact on one's capacity to locomote in space. Army-crawling on the floor is a precursor to walking, where the head continually counterspirals against the working spiral. The same goes for walking, where the focus remains forward while the torso and limbs counterspiral below. Bringing your awareness to your arms gives you information about your tendencies, such as whether they both swing as you walk, each taking its turn in Primary and Secondary alternately. You may notice that one arm moves quite a bit while the other stays relatively still. You can also notice whether you tend to overly spiral the upper body and not spiral the lower, or vice versa.

Video: Walking with Primary and Secondary Spirals

It is also possible to look at walking through the Primary, Secondary, and Reset model. Extending a leg forward is a Primary action, and as you step on that leg, your overall spine will extend through your standing leg, which becomes a Secondary, which will Reset just as you are done propelling yourself with it. This process repeats itself rhythmically as you continue to walk.

Pushing a full shopping cart—the resistance of the cart's weight is useful in this exploration—is a good vehicle for observing the relationship of the arms to the hips, legs, and feet in walking. Is your weight transferring easily from one foot to the other? Paying attention to the pressure of the hands on the handle, can you feel how one hand is pushing while the other is Resetting? If you can feel this, pay attention to the rhythmic exchange between the upper and lower Engagements. Do you prefer standing on one leg more than another? Or both? It is important to allow the shoulders and hips to work together in concert, which is transferable to assisted walking with a walker, cane, or crutch.

Sawing

Interestingly, sawing a piece of wood is essentially the same as crawling or pushing the grocery cart. The sawing motion of the arm is the one we tend to notice most, but the legs and the hand holding the piece of wood are also at play, alternately Engaging and Resetting, which allows the sawing to take place. In the instance of the harder labor of sawing, the non-sawing arm/hand stabilizes the piece of wood, giving you three points of support. With three points of support, it is easier to feel spirals and their Engagements and Resets. This idea might also be applied to less strenuous tasks, like using a knife to slice bread or brushing your teeth. Notice whether you tend to hold the whole body rigidly against the sawing arm, preventing yourself from spiraling. Then try to find Upper and Lower Engagements and Resets, and slowly feel the rhythm in your limbs and the *ball* direction. This needs to be more of an investigation than trying to do it right.

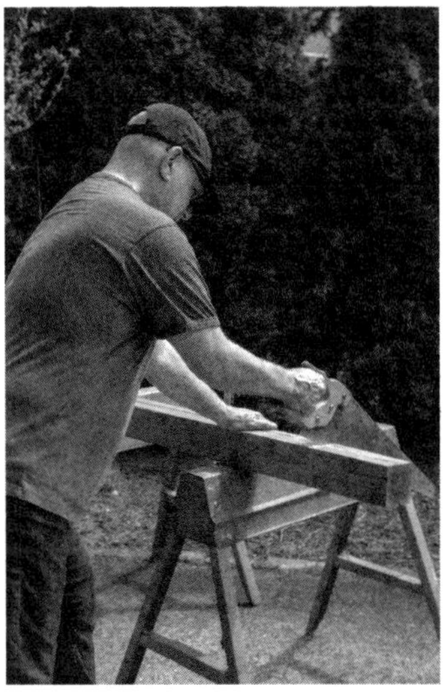

Chopping

Wielding an axe to chop wood, and other similar types of activities, can be observed from the Integrated Model. As you face the log on a stump in front of you, aiming to split it with the axe, the *ball* would be going back in an *Ocean* phase, arms supporting the trunk with the legs free. If you then pass the axe over your right side, you can lengthen your right hand on the handle and transfer your weight onto the right foot (spiraling action), with the left hand relating to the right leg in Primary and the *ball* escaping left. Once the axe passes behind you, the right hand and arm become Secondary, the weight shifts on both legs and the *ball* is now going forward (*Seagulls* into *Beach Chair*), with the head released at the top of the spine, eyes starting to look down. As you start to wield the axe in its last arc, the *ball* shifts backward (*Sandals*) while both hands are now together and the axe is splitting the log. Notice the clear switch in activity within the arms from holding the axe behind you in an arch (*Seagulls*/arms Engage) to swinging the axe forward (*Sandals*/arms Reset). Usually, there is a tendency to hold the axe too strongly, instead of sometimes letting the hips power the activity and other times letting the arms Engage fully. We will look at such Complex and Integrated Models in sports in the next section.

Video: Hammer

Drinking from a Glass

While drinking water, it can be fun to notice the interchanging of Engagements and Resets in the hand while holding a glass of water. Sitting facing the glass on the table, start to pick it up toward your mouth. As you tip the glass toward your lips, notice the Engagement transfer toward the thumb. And as you put it back down, feel the pressure change toward your fingers while your thumb Resets. This is the simple truth about our bodies: They constantly change in activity. There is no "holding" a glass of water, only an exchange of Engagements and Resets!

Recreational Sports: Introduction

In professional sports, many directives are aimed at shaving off a second, gaining an inch, building specific strength or flexibility around a part of the body, or doing whatever it takes to attain the competitive goal. This attitude often bleeds into recreational sports, causing everyday athletes to become confused as to why they are doing one training protocol over another (sometimes the same can be said of professional athletes). We aim to support athletes, pro or amateur, at any age and any stage of development. Regardless of the sport you are engaging in, it is important to question coaching ideas that trickle down from professional sports settings and prioritize understanding your habits and adaptations so that you can continue to refine your technique, appropriate to your age and level of skill. Often, someone hangs up their skis or their bike if they think it is the activity itself that is causing pain. Weekend warrior athletes who have had a considerable amount of physical therapy might stop participating in their sport rather than considering how they use their bodies. For example, if your knees are hurting while running, you might think that switching to bike riding is a safe alternative; however, you are likely to find that switching to another sport may not solve the issue, since the way you used your body in one thing will likely be replicated in another.

Sports

Some sports relate obviously to the Simple Model. In swimming, the breaststroke is easily observed as symmetrical and can be understood as a Secondary pull of the arms followed by the head diving into the water in a Primary powered by the legs. The same swim stroke could benefit from being investigated through the Integrated Model, either with the *ball* activity (*ball forward* in the pull of the arms) or with the Upper and Lower Triangles, where the Upper is engaged in the pull and Resets when the legs are Engaging. In a butterfly stroke, similar patterns are present. Diving off a diving board, we can see the Four Phases at play: The pressure on the board is a *Beach Chair* phase, propelling off the board relates to a *Sandals* phase, flying in the air in an arch toward the water is an *Ocean* phase, while entering the water is a *Seagull* phase. We have all probably observed a child trying to enter the water with the *ball going back* only to end up splatting on the surface of the water or applying pressure on the springboard with their *ball going back* and seeing them abort the takeoff. Antagonistic action in the pelvis is very important in the control of diving and other aerial sports. Adding a somersault to the dive adds an extra series of phases to the activity, either in Primary or Secondary. And adding twists quickly brings us into the Complex Model.

Additional symmetrical activities include rowing with two oars (sculling), sailing on a one-person boat, and wheelchair racing, where we also find correlations with either the Simple or Integrated Model. Rowing in particular has a strong affinity to the Four Phases on the ball, including the use of the limbs. Any sailboat going up against a strong wind will see the sailor lean out, sending the *ball* toward the center of the boat. If the wind lags, the *ball* right away starts to go backward. Wheelchair racing, when propelled by a strong push out and down, sees the *ball* going backward, and between pushes the *ball* Resets forward. For all these activities, staying stuck in one or two phases will quickly be detrimental. Do not be fooled by the shape of the body. In leaning back in space to counter the pull of the wind, even if the shape of the body seems to be in Primary, consider the movement of the *ball* (forward) and where the Engagement actually is (Lower Triangle). As the wind dies down a bit, the *ball* goes back and the head comes forward, with the body's shape not having changed much. And yet, the first movement is a *Seagulls* phase with the second a *Sandals* phase. Similar thinking applies to the wheelchair racer, where the push of the wheels is in a *Sandals* phase and the Reset is in a *Seagulls* phase. Being able to notice where the *ball* is meant to move and how we habitually interfere with the activity will help redirect toward better use, with more enjoyment and less pain.

Doing free throws in basketball can be seen from the lens of Primary and Secondary. Looking down as you dribble the basketball is a Primary. Finding the power of the Engagement in Primary by sending the imaginary *ball* back will help clarify the use of that moment. Holding the basketball in your hands and looking at the basket, you can be in either an *Ocean* phase or *Beach Chair* phase. In tossing the basketball, your imaginary *ball* will go forward as you aim to be in a *Seagulls* phase. The toss of the ball toward the basket is a spiral. Bringing the elbows in encourages stability in Primary in the Upper Triangle, allowing the Lower Triangle to extend itself fully.

Kayaking is a particularly beautiful example of the Complex Model, with the spirals continually switching from side to side. Reviewing Movement Exploration 7.4 on the ball, leaning from side to side will help decipher habits in relation to kayaking. It is fun to notice that the kayak is flying forward because your pelvis (Lower Triangle) is Resetting forward, in support of the arms' Engagement against the water (*Seagulls* into *Beach Chair*). When kayaking becomes an integrated activity, the rhythmic coordination of sending the *ball* forward to propel the kayak generates a sense of competence and enjoyment.

Running (as well as walking), from a movement pattern perspective, is very similar to kayaking. Cyclic spirals propel the body forward in space. The only difference is that the kayaker rarely goes uphill (up a waterfall) and usually has the advantage of an even terrain, unless they find themselves in whitewater, waterfalls, or rapids. Running can be done on flat, even surfaces but also usually includes uphill and downhill terrain. If a kayak is going down a small waterfall, the *ball* would be going generally forward. Similarly, if you were to run downhill, the *ball* can be consciously redirected forward in either B*each Chair* or *Seagulls,* and as you run or walk uphill, the only difference is the change in Upper and Lower Engagements. It is important to remind yourself that you can always send the ball in another direction. For example, going uphill with the *ball* back will automatically call for either an *Ocean* or *Sandals* phase—perhaps not the usual. Try to imagine looking uphill while sending the *ball* back, or running downhill looking down on the floor while sending the *ball* forward. How do those choices feel? These options are disaffined with the task at hand.

Adjusting your bicycle when it comes to where you sit to pedal can benefit your body mechanics. Some bikes are reclined, with the pedals in front and above the pelvis, others are city bikes where you are seated upright, and others have you inclined over the front handlebars. In the reclining bike, you are perfectly placed to be in a Primary Ball Forward (*Beach Chair*) phase. The Engagement of the upper back on the seat back frees your legs to pedal. If your bicycle sits you more upright, in general your hips will be Engaging and your arms freeing. The *ball* will

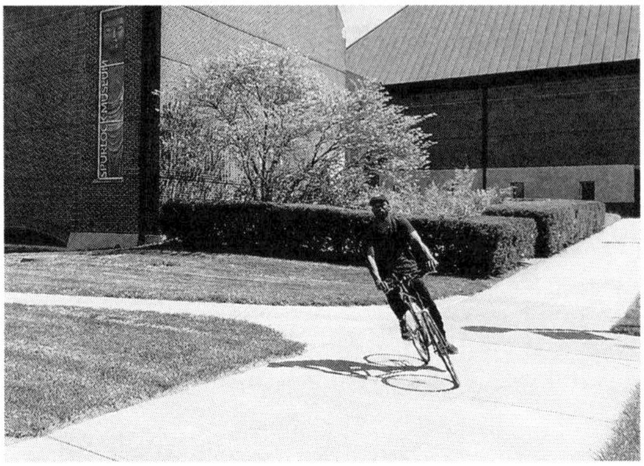

As cyclist turns the corner, his head leads into the turn and the imaginary ball escapes away.

be encouraged forward or back depending on surface levels and when your bike accelerates or decelerates. If your bike inclines you over the handlebars, there will be a tendency for your hips (Lower Triangle) to be freer as your arms (Upper Triangle) Engage during your ride. Also, the cyclic activity encourages shifts of weight from side to side as well as changes in Engagement from Upper to Lower. If the weight is transferring, then you know spirals are present. Turning a corner will easily facilitate the action of the *ball* while the head leans into the turn. In all setups, going uphill or downhill will also reveal the activity of the *ball*. You can search for the subtle Engagements and Resets. Pushing on the pedals or the handlebars is an Engagement that is usually accompanied by a Reset. Bike shops will fit your bike to you to facilitate proper mechanics, but ultimately, it is up to you to observe and interact with the movement patterns of the Framework. Motorcycles and mopeds are like bicycles and will constantly give you feedback on your approach to keeping yourself balanced. Stationary bicycles will not give you much feedback in terms of spirals or *ball* activity.

Video: Riding the Bike

Immediately after our zoom class on Friday, I got on my bicycle. As I was riding towards campus, I noticed a new awareness of my body: the secondary curve of my upper back accompanied by a slight pull on the handlebars, and a primary curve that felt more pronounced and supportive than usual through my lower back and pelvis as my feet pushed toward the pedals. My handlebars are high, almost cruiser-style, so I'm usually aware of the upward posture and secondary curve through my upper body, but I think in the past I've overcorrected the curve through my lower back and tried to make a matching secondary curve, placing my whole spine into one big arched semicircle. By allowing and encouraging the natural primary curve I felt, I think I can find more ease on my bicycle (which will be welcome, as my primary—pun intended—mode of transportation).

—Anna Peretz Rogovoy, Dance graduate student, University of Illinois

Skiing, whether downhill on snow or pulled by a boat on water, promotes the embodiment of spirals and all phases of the *ball*. When going straight down the ski hill or pulled by a boat, if standing up tall, the *ball* would need to be directed forward. On the hill, if you wanted to speed up and incline yourself forward, the *ball* would start to go back (*Ocean*) but would eventually Reset itself into either a *Seagulls* or *Beach Chair* phase. As you start to want to turn, the head leads the spiral (as in Movement Exploration 5.3) and, aided by the pull of the arms, results in the body turning sideways either in the water or on the snow. At all times, you are paying attention to keeping the *ball* toward the direction of the pull (either the boat or gravity).

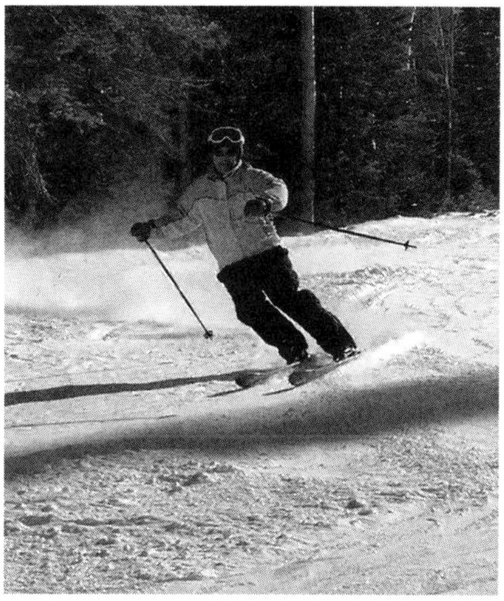

Video: Skiing

Notice the change in leg activity from one side to the other, where the leg toward the bottom of the hill automatically goes into pronation, while the uphill leg goes into supination. In the weight shift to the other side, the legs Reset and then switch roles—the pronating leg providing push and power while the supinating leg gradually frees to direct the next action. This pattern can be found in cross-country skate skiing, rollerblading, roller skating, and ice skating. In contrast, imagine someone starting to ski, always keeping their legs Engaged in Primary with their skis in a "V" (with front tips of skis pointing in) and sense how difficult it would be to turn with both legs staying equally Engaged. To rhythmically switch from one side to the other, the weight needs to transfer from the outside ski, freeing up the uphill ski so that the arms can lead the change and the second ski can follow the direction. When using ski poles, it is easier to engage your arms in the transfer of weight. Clear feedback from the upper body and gravity can stimulate the legs to Reset (as in Movement Exploration 8.2).

This is a good moment to reconsider swimming in terms of the crawling stroke. A cursory look at people swimming this stroke in the pool will reveal a lot of pulling themselves along the surface, mostly facing the bottom of the pool, except for the moment of twisting their necks to inhale. Often the upper back and arms stay in a Primary pattern while the lower back arches, forcing the pelvis and legs more toward Secondary. Instead, at its core, the crawl is a spiraling activity. So rather than continually keeping your body facing toward the bottom of the pool, allow yourself to spiral fully, rolling from side to side. When pulling through the water, you are in an *Ocean* phase, extended with the *ball* back (to the ceiling or sky). For instance, if you are pulling with your right hand, this helps transfer the weight onto your left side, which lengthens the reach of your left arm to release your right hand out of the water. This sequencing allows for a glide on your side before the next action—you will recognize the side activity as similar to Movement Exploration 9.3—leaning sideways with the *ball* escaping to the opposite side, in this case toward the ceiling or sky. The sequence repeats, alternating sides and

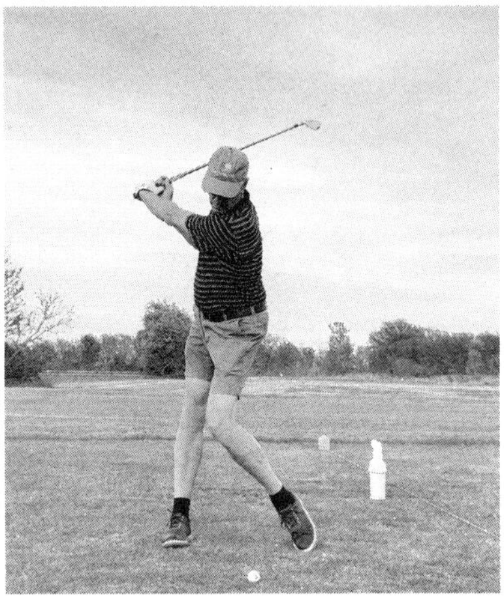

An Engaged spiral

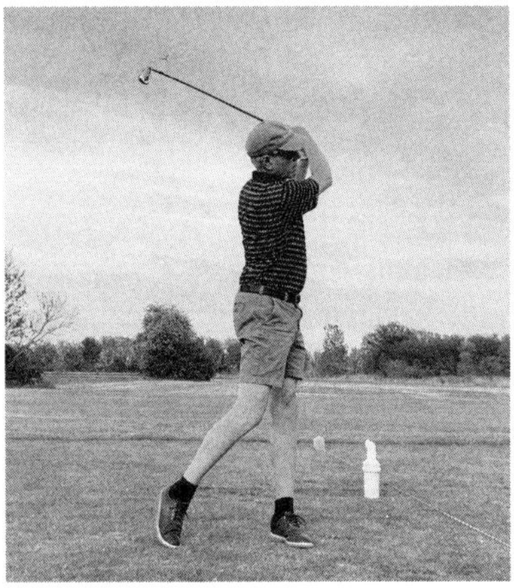

A Reset

allowing for Resetting in between strokes. In this version of the crawl, the arms do most of the work. The beating of the legs serves as support and does not overtake the head and arms. And if you try it, you will notice that any pushing of the hips (*ball*) or lower back in Secondary will only cause you to sink toward the bottom.[2]

Golf lends itself well to analysis via the Framework. The traditional images of a golfer inclined over a ball or having just hit the ball, finishing in a full spiral, fully express the sport's range of movement. As you incline over the ball to putt or prepare to swing, knowing your habitual tendencies can be informative. Do you normally send the *ball* back in an *Ocean* phase, do you prefer sending the *ball* forward, or do you simply try not to move your pelvis at all? Typically, you will see a beginning golfer raise their club ready to hit, and then in the swing, hesitate to use their Lower Triangle to power up their arms. It appears that they are trying to hit the golf ball solely with their arms, instead of the arms being a result of the spiraling action of the hips and spine.

As a right-handed golfer raises their arms to hit the ball, the left shoulder will be in Primary, in a counter spiral to the head (eyes looking at the golf ball). We could call this a "loaded" spiral—the left shoulder to the transferred weight on the right leg is in a powerfully loaded Primary. Releasing this "wound up" power in the next phase of the swing is the Reset, which, if not interfered with, sends the ball toward the intended direction. Inside this seemingly simple action, thinking about weight shifting, spirals, *ball* direction, and Upper/Lower Triangles are all possible. In putting, the same patterns are present in smaller, subtler variations.

Video: Golf

The same movement dynamics apply to hitting a baseball, so much so that if a golf coach thinks a beginner is having good luck hitting with power, they will often ask if the person has played baseball or softball. The weight transfer of the hips and legs, to power up the arms and then land again in the hips and legs, is a skill that needs timing and freedom, beautiful when it happens, hard to fix if interfered with. A similar skill is needed in hitting a tennis ball, wiffle ball, or birdie in playing badminton. The moment of hitting the object occurs when the arms/Upper Triangle Engage and the hips/Lower Triangle Reset, followed immediately by the reverse. In Western culture, when sitting or standing, there is a general tendency to always

Engage the hips/Lower Triangle, never completely letting them go. Playing a sport that allows for feedback with the Engagement of the Upper Triangle gives you a chance to let go of any extra work with the hips.

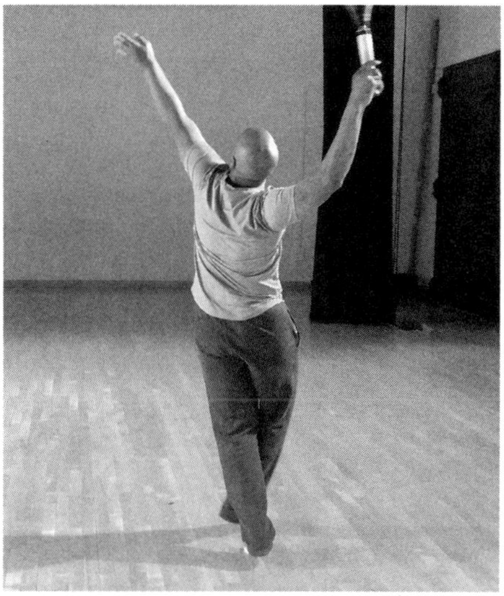

The Lower Triangle powering the Upper Triangle before a serve

Video: Tennis

To see another example of a beautiful spiral, watch people who bowl. The skill, especially at the end of the throw, will reveal a simple balanced spiral, with the throwing hand and the forward foot in Primary while the other two limbs are in Secondary. A further spiral in the throwing hand usually makes the ball spin. Compare the end position in bowling to golfing. Can you see the resemblance?

Riding a horse used to be a common sight in our communities, in the countrysides, and in cities. The activity is now relegated to expensive sports such as racing, show jumping, hunting, polo, and dressage. The care and riding of horses is also used in various therapeutic settings. There is a reciprocal relationship between the horse's movement and the way the rider communicates with the horse through their thoughts and movements, which help them come back in proper relationship with their own body movements. Horses have a few phases (gaits) of their own, such as the walk, canter, trot, and gallop. Thinking that a person could hold themselves rigidly upright on a moving horse can be quickly debunked by riding one. Watching a rodeo where a horse and rider might catch a bull, circle barrels, handle cattle, or compete to see which of the two can outlast the other will prove the point. A rider must be at ease and able to adapt at all moments. In the rodeo example, it is fairly easy to see the need for a well-adapted pelvis action (*ball*) in relationship with the head. No planning will do—only a free, adaptive body can meet the demands of the bucking horse (or bull!). In a horse race, we can observe the way a jockey needs to transfer weight from their arms to their legs on the horse. The rocking on the horse is an *Ocean* phase to a *Beach Chair* phase. In a more everyday ride, the rider will need to be able to either transfer their weight onto the working front leg of the horse (with the *ball* going in a forward diagonal—*semi Beach Chair* phase) or allow all phases to be at play in a trot. Arms are not to continually pull the reins, nor are they completely inactive, and it is the same for the legs. Riding a horse is a wonderful opportunity to let go of the movement patterns that interfere with the use of the horse.

Some sports require a lot of power, such as boxing, martial arts, and American football, among others. In general, the power experienced at the end of a hit is a Primary activity. Finding all the Primaries (see Chapter Four) throughout the body will help unleash the strength of Primary in a punch or a body hit while keeping the legs light. The skill is in releasing just enough out of Primary to extend the arm in Secondary to punch and then Reset. This is usually best done in an *Ocean* phase, unless we are dealing with an uppercut, which will require a *Seagull* phase. In contrast, a hook will send the *ball* sideways, away from the direction of the punch. This is illustrated by a quote from famed boxer Muhammad Ali: "float like a butterfly, sting like a bee." An informed use of spirals will also elicit power. For people who habitually solicit Secondary for strength, Primary usually comes as a relief, as a centering force. Finding Primary power, as seen in a grounded Sumo wrestler or a karate martial artist who is about to break a plank, might feel unusual to most people unless they were to emphatically pound their fist on a table while saying "that's enough!"

Physical Training

Physical training, including strength, flexibility, and cross-training, provides many opportunities for applying the Framework. In this context, it is especially important to recognize your relationship to gravity, and to discover which movement patterns would be most useful to support the exercise that you are doing. For example, pulling handles situated above your head will take on a different meaning if you are looking up at the handles versus if you are looking down. In lat pulldowns, while sitting and holding on to the bar, it's important to remember the movement exploration of pulling yourself along the floor (Movement Exploration 4.3). First, from the Simple Model, consider that you begin by releasing your arms to the bar in a gentle Primary from your hip joint to your palms and that the pull is a Secondary. From the Integrated Model, you begin in a *Beach Chair* phase and then, as you start to look up, you transition into a *Seagulls* phase. Keep in mind that as the arms pull, the shoulder girdle releases along the direction of the pull, ultimately allowing the trunk to lengthen. This should help avoid crunching into the lower back, accentuating the lower back's secondary curve. In general, attempting to leave the gaze in "neutral" will most likely lead to your habits running unchecked—visual intention clarifies overall body patterning.

Consider the bench press. From the Simple Model, lying on your back already encourages you toward a Secondary pattern. And yet, the push of the weight(s) calls for a strong Primary. It will be important to notice whether the bench height supports you going into a Primary. Putting a towel under your head might also help stop any extra, unneeded Secondary in the head/neck area. While pushing the weight up, keep the overall Primary alive by sending your back into the bench. From an Integrated Model, pushing the weight engages the Upper Triangle and Resets the Lower Triangle, freeing up the pelvis and legs. Lying on your back, before pushing the weight toward the ceiling, is an *Ocean* phase, with the arms active and the *ball* going back toward the bench. The pushing of the weight itself transitions into a *Beach Chair* phase, with the *ball* releasing toward the ceiling as the lower continues to Reset. When the weight is up toward the ceiling, can you wiggle your knees, move your legs, and feel the freedom in your neck? A bench press is an inverted version of Movement Exploration 8.2: Rocking Back and Forth on All Fours.

Some forms of physical training have specialized equipment, such as Pilates, Gyrokinesis, and TRX training, among others. In working with equipment, it is always important to consider the intent behind the movement to see if your movement pattern is a match for the activity. For example, the Pilates Reformer Footwork series has you lying on your back on the reformer rolling platform and extending your legs to various degrees. In these exercises, be aware that lying supine with your knees bent and your head on a bolster will encourage the Secondaries (low back and neck) in your body to release toward Primary, while stimulating the Primary of the thoracic region toward a Secondary. Usually, lying on your back is more of a Secondary, but on the reformer with knees and head forward, you find yourself in a Primary. The legs' extension takes you toward a Secondary and, as such, allows the legs and shoulder girdle to rotate slightly outwardly. In that same Footwork exercise, still on the reformer, consider whether you are using your Lower Triangle to power the push of the carriage up along the machine and if so, whether your arms are Resetting. Ask yourself where the *ball* should go and what phase of activity you believe yourself to be in. In theory, if your Lower is Engaged and your body is extending in space, you would be in the *Seagulls* phase. And then, to release your legs coming back, see if thinking about your arms will help you Reset your legs to the original position, ending in a *Beach Chair* phase (legs Reset). In the same manner, if you are using your arms at any time on the reformer, see if your legs can Reset some.

Doing a squat with a kettlebell accentuates the need to fully Engage the Upper Triangle to completely free the legs. In getting out of the squat, the activity switches and the legs power up the extension, while the arms Reset even as they are holding a weight. When holding a weight, Resets become a matter of contrast rather than a feeling of release or freedom. The freedom is in the antagonistic action present between the Upper and Lower Triangles. A similar situation is present when you spiral the kettlebell from a squat to one leg with the opposing arm coming across, similar to a punch up into the air. The transfer of weight engages the leg and the arm on that same side, which leaves the thrusting arm and leg of the same side in a Reset.

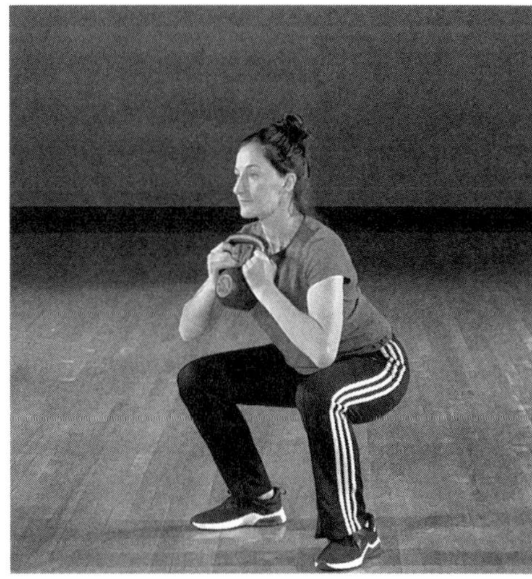

Video: Kettlebell

Abdominal workouts usually include crunches. Thinking about direction in abdominal work allows for a freer hip and spine relationship during the workout. First, it is useful to experience doing crunches on a physioball, consciously allowing the ball to move. In the Framework, coming forward into a "crunch," you would send the ball back, with the feet engaging or grounding against the floor. By doing this, you prevent the shoulders from jamming into the trunk/hips. You are in a *Sandals* phase. Returning from there, you would allow the ball to go forward. Once you have experienced this on an actual ball, you can try it on a mat, just thinking about the ball directions.

Reflections

Human nature is to look for the right way to do something and to hold on to it once found. Be wary of cementing the proposed ideas as hard, fast rules. Keep in mind that some of what you are habitually doing might be great for you. The three models are there mainly to help you discern among all the ideas out there and what works best for you.

As stated at the beginning of this chapter, the act of continually paying attention can be exhausting, both physically and mentally. It's important to rest after paying attention to your patterns in a way that allows the whole of you to digest the information, ready for another exploration.

It is also important to point out that pain is often the motivator for seeking new methods for performing daily activities. If that is the case, first be sure you have explored all medical options. The Framework is not a replacement for proper medical attention. At all times, be gentle with yourself and take a lot of time resting before, during, and after any attempts at redirecting activity. If pain shows up or increases, back off, and spend time doing less and thinking about the directions more. Take smaller steps. Climb stairs on all fours. Put your hands on the bed before getting out of bed in the morning. Use a chair in front of you to get up from sitting. Always look to make the activity simpler and clearer in relationship to intent. Never think that pushing through will give you any lasting results. And never give up aligning intent with activity as an exploration that can lessen pain.

Finally, you might notice a tendency to think that the way we live every day has little impact on our bodies, as if we were made of rock. But, just like a dry plant's drooping leaves will perk up after a proper watering, at any age, our body can dramatically change almost immediately if we simply stop doing the unneeded and disaffined effort. It can feel as if change in daily routines and activities takes a lot of work—the weight of our habits and fixed ideas can be hard on us and take time to open up. Yet our bodies and minds are designed to be adaptive and resilient, and the tools of the Framework can provide that needed space for considering our choices. At any time, you can circle back to very clear and simple approaches or dive into challenging complexities. The choices are yours!

NOTES

1. Constructive Rest Position was first described by Lulu Sweigard in *Human Movement Potential: Its Ideokinetic Facilitation* (see bibliography).
2. This approach to swimming is influenced by the work of Steven Shaw, author of *The Art of Swimming: A New Direction using the Alexander Technique.*

Chapter 15

Guest Contributions—Dance, Movement, and Acting Applications

How can one apply Framework principles to ballroom dance, Argentine Tango, pole and aerial dancing, acting, or teaching dance fitness in a gym setting? Contributors share their experiences and offer examples to illustrate their discoveries.

Framework for Integration and Acting

Jacque Lynn Bell

I have enjoyed teaching Movement and the Alexander Technique to the Actor Training Program at the University of Utah for the last three decades. Although it has always been fulfilling, my enjoyment and the students' transformations have increased tremendously over the last several years as I have had the amazing opportunity to be exposed to and engage in more in-depth study in Framework for Integration.

Framework for Integration invites a three-dimensionality that was lacking in my teaching previously. I don't mean this in a vague metaphorical sense; I mean this literally. Instead of focusing on lengthening and widening, as a more classical training in the Alexander Technique might encourage, the concepts of Primary and Secondary from the Framework allow for depth, spiraling, and a greater ability for freedom of movement in every direction.

As a student enters my studio for their private lesson, I can see their general tendencies in how they are using their bodies in terms of Primary and Secondary. Often the actors will have been coached to pull their shoulders back and push their chest out, leaving them to go about their lives in a continual Secondary. Although I know it is done with best intentions, both on the part of the teacher and the student, it can affect performance and be exhausting. And, as I point out to the students, if they are already in Secondary, they have nowhere further to go. For example, if they want to emphasize their shock, confidence, or outrage, they are already fully extended, and there is no way to increase the expression of those emotions. And if they walk around with their torso already in Primary, their ability to portray a character who suddenly becomes sad, protective, or introverted is extremely limited. As the student becomes aware of their preferences and the possibilities for using Primary, Secondary, and Reset to express themselves, their range increases tremendously.

Understanding Primary, Secondary, and Reset is an easy means for the actors to choose softening in the neck, chest, pelvis, or knees, or extension of the same. As I guide them to try Primary, Secondary, or Reset while they are giving their monologue, they are enlightened by the possibilities and the way their subtle changes in body language affect their emotions.

Using the foundation of inhibition in general, as the actor is giving their monologue, I use the Framework to direct them. I might say, "Try allowing your upper body to move toward Secondary as your pelvis releases into Primary." Then, I might follow up with, "Allow that to Reset as your right shoulder subtly spirals into Secondary and your left side gently moves towards Primary." Or "Reset that and invite your head to release away from the top of your spine as your neck goes into Primary, and then very slowly Reset that and let the neck lengthen into Secondary as the head releases forward and up." As the lesson continues, I let them choose where to use Primary, Secondary, and Reset.

By the end of the lesson, my student will usually respond something to this effect, often with tears in their eyes, "This gives me so many more choices! I had no idea that I could perform these lines in Primary, and as a consequence, I would feel gentle and vulnerable where I used to feel stiff and unconnected. Or that I could do this other section in Secondary and feel strong and defensive, which gives my character much more depth. My emotions are more available, my breathing is easier, and my voice is coming from a deeper place within me. I am excited to use these skills in my acting class!"

I am continually amazed by how the simple access to Primary, Secondary, and Reset dramatically changes the acting. Although I always think what great actors my students are as they initially give their monologue, after they apply the Framework, I am no longer outside of the action judging the actor; I am pulled in, deeply moved, often to tears myself.

Jacque Lynn Bell is a dancer/choreographer and AmSAT certified teacher of the Alexander Technique. She received her MFA in Choreography at the University of Utah, where she has taught movement and the Alexander Technique in the Department of Theater for over thirty years. For the past seven years, she has had the opportunity to study the Framework with Luc Vanier and Elizabeth Johnson and has been thrilled to integrate it into everything she does.

Teaching a Dance Fitness Class: Embedding Principles of the Framework

Rebecca Nettl-Fiol

Teaching a dance class aimed at cardio fitness in a gym setting, where the norm is to follow the instructor without stopping to explain, is quite different from teaching a dance technique class, where the expectation is to give information about *how* to do the movement. I have been teaching a dance fitness class for over ten years, populated mainly by women aged forty-five or older. Similar to Zumba, the class is fifty minutes of nonstop dancing derived from popular forms like salsa, merengue, Bollywood, swing, and hip-hop, set to a variety of music styles. My challenge is finding ways of bringing my dance knowledge and principles from the Framework to the students within the context of this type of class, where participants vary in age, movement ability, and longevity in terms of their participation in the class.

My greatest wish is to share my joy of dancing to music, while offering basic movement principles that invite the students to fully engage with their whole selves—body, mind, and spirit. Each of the twelve dances that make up a class is choreographed so that it really feels like a dance, with a degree of complexity that challenges but hopefully doesn't discourage. I carefully weave my playlist with contrasts in genres, tempos, and rhythmic structures, with a prerequisite that each song I select compels me to get up and move! To me, there is nothing more joyful than being immersed in a room full of people dancing together. To that end, I add times when we interact. Rather than always facing front, I may choose to do a circle dance, or I may ask students to partner up or to move about the space and intermingle with different people as they dance.

In creating the movement material for the class, I always consider how I am using Primary, Secondary, and Reset, such that we don't get stuck in one or the other but find ways to alternate or fluctuate between them. I don't talk about the theory behind it; I simply build it into the dance phrases and then encourage them to experience the fullness of each, through my demonstration and shouting out cues, like "open" and "close" or "in" and "out." Or I might point out that you can fully reach into the space, for example, and then simply let that energy go, which propels you to go in a different direction. It is exciting to see a whole class of people opening

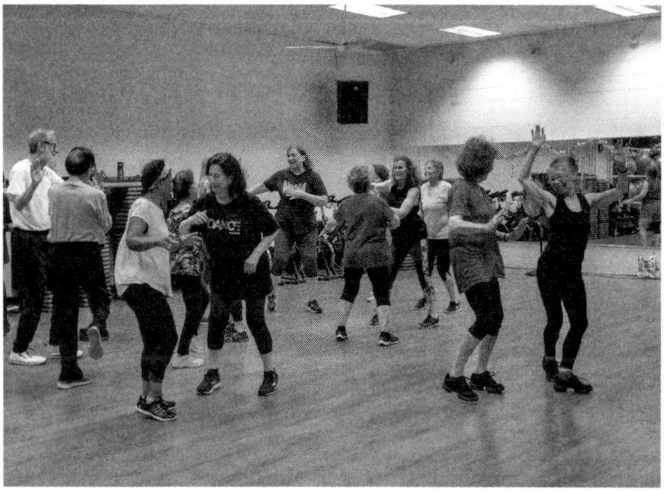

their faces and chests to the sky, the experience of an ecstatic moment, contrasted by a softening into self before reaching out into the world again.

The same goes for spirals. Latin dances are especially conducive to engaging and resetting spirals. To encourage this, I do my best to clearly demonstrate and even show with my hands how the Primary spiral can shorten and then Reset to switch to the other spiral. I also use rhythm to stimulate this action of Reset, so that if you do the proper phrasing, you are most likely to discover the mechanics I am looking for. Phrasing is always at the forefront when I'm making up the dances, when I consider how one movement leads to another in a rhythmic way. I stay away from bland or even timing in favor of more complex rhythmic structures that encourage a particular coordination.

Cueing as we go, briefly demonstrating a new step, or being aware of what I am emphasizing as I lead the class are all ways to encourage concepts that are directly or indirectly related to the Framework. Again, I try to model full-out, joyful dancing, so that I am smiling much of the time and having fun myself. Then, I encourage the students to extend the movement through their whole body and self, not just arms or legs. To me, it is never just about steps, even though the steps may be challenging to learn. But how is the rest of the body also a part of the step?

I continually encourage resilience. I want them to find the bounce inside of the step—how can you rebound from one step to another, using the elastic energy in the muscles? I also emphasize the upbeat that comes before the downbeat, using it for a breath or an "up" movement. And for the arm movements, I offer reasons for the gestures, so they are connected to the body and the meaning of the movement. Movement intention is key. For example, for an arm gesture that swipes strongly across the front of the body, I ask them to beat a rug like they are cleaning it; or if we are making a half turn and walking, I might ask them to turn away from someone they don't want to be with anymore and walk away. These kinds of motivations stimulate a full-body response. I also give cues for where to focus or how the eyes can lead a movement.

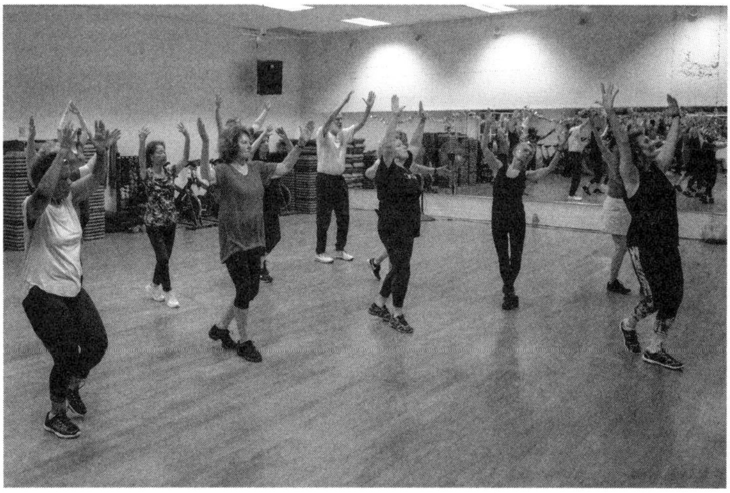

Embedding the Framework principles in the movement phrases, demonstrating what I hope to convey, shouting out cues, and sometimes taking an extra minute to explain a movement concept, are the means I use for providing insights into an enhanced movement/dance experience in my dance fitness classes. It is my hope that the folks who take my classes get an inadvertent lesson in the Framework that will carry over into their everyday lives.

Rebecca Nettl-Fiol, coauthor of *Dance and the Alexander Technique: Exploring the Missing Link* and *The Body Electric: Evolving Practices in Dance Training*, is a professor of Dance at the University of Illinois Urbana-Champaign, and an AmSAT certified teacher of the Alexander Technique. In her long tenure at the university, she has designed and implemented many courses in the dance science and somatics field, and she continues to research the integration of the Alexander Technique and the Framework principles into her teaching in all contexts. In addition, she has developed and taught a dance fitness class in the community for more than a decade.

Framework for Integration Applied to Argentine Tango Dancing

Christopher Neville

I'd like to suggest some possible uses of the Framework in tango, starting with Engagements and Resets, then Primary and Secondary, and finally Upper and Lower Triangles. Before we start, a few words about tango. Tango is a dance of opposites—an interplay of opposing forces that can be more or less harmonious and balanced in alternating polarities. A fundamental reason the Framework is so valuable to tango is because it also is a system based on various polarities. These are not just differences or variations, but actual opposites—binary options that create oscillating, alternating actions.

With that in mind, let's move on to the first polarity, Engage and Reset. In tango, this easily applies to the legs, as in the difference between the standing and free leg. If the standing leg is Engaged, the free leg is Reset. When there is confusion about the exchange of Engagements and Resets, it often results in an overall lack of freedom and support; the standing leg might not support the weight confidently and the free leg might hold onto ideas of grounding instead of fully freeing. Engagements and Rests also exist in the arms and hands. I've known good dancers who are never able to Reset the embrace, which can lead to all sorts of shoulder tension and pain. Engagements and Resets also relate to musicality in the dancers' ability to speed up and slow down the dance. Without being able to Engage part of a musical phrase (for example, speed up) and then Reset to ride the flow of the rest of the phrase (perhaps unwinding to slow down and pause), most dancers have a hard time playing the full spectrum and consequently have a very narrow range of musicality.

The next polarity is Primary and Secondary. Here, an extremely valuable lesson is the antagonistic action that exists in the tango. When dancing face to face in close embrace, the partners are doing opposite things. One person is walking forward, while the other person is walking backward. When you understand a forward step as more toward an overall Primary and a back step as more toward overall

Secondary, you can effectively counter your partner with the opposite activity. The language of Primary and Secondary helps us find a wider range of movement and to understand where both support and reach are coming from. The Primary and Secondary relationships exist in our individual bodies and movement habits—those possibilities multiply within the couple's dynamic.

The last thing is the attention to the Upper and Lower Triangles, which I see as being active in both the embrace and the step. How the lead communicates and transmits direction through to the follower's feet is a function of the Upper and Lower Triangles. The first thing to notice is how the Upper Triangle can create connection in the embrace that Resets and frees up the legs. When the Upper Triangle is "loaded" with support, the lower body is more mobile. Where it gets interesting is when we look at halves of the body and include an attention to spirals. When one side of the leader's embrace is Engaging with one side of the follower's embrace, both partners' standing and free legs give the couple a balanced way to power *ochos* (a fundamental tango step that involves pivoting on one foot/leg, swiveling the hips, and stepping across the midline with the other—a figure-eight patterning that can repeat as many times as the dancers want). The stability and support of the "standing leg arm" allows an easy extension of the free leg. With this interplay between support and freedom, the dancers can push the spirals inherent in tango to their beautiful fullness.

Using the tools of the Framework gives us a fluid, controlled, soft and strong, graceful and powerful dance. The Framework tools can help prevent the all-too-common problems tango dancers face and offer a pathway and a pedagogy to reduce often experienced confusion and disconnect between partners. If you have a tango experience that includes a frustrating combination of lurching, stumbling, knee knocking, and beyond, looking into Framework applications can really enlighten and clarify. I now use the Framework as a fundamental tool in my tango teaching and have seen a transformative difference in my students as well as my own dancing.

Christopher Neville is an artist, entrepreneur, and AmSat certified teacher of the Alexander Technique. He was educated in the apprenticeship style with a couple of artists and craftsmen before discovering the Alexander Technique in 2005 and becoming a certified teacher in 2020. In 2019 he cofounded Two Flame Tango, a somatic tango school in Salt Lake City, where he currently serves as a program designer and primary instructor.

Framework for Integration: A New Approach to Teaching Ballroom Dancing

Alex Tecza

In 2011, my partner and I gave a demonstration and lecture at the University of Illinois Urbana-Champaign. After our performance, Becky Nettl-Fiol struck up a conversation with us, telling us how much of what we showed and talked about went very much in line with her research she had been conducting with Luc Vanier and Elizabeth Johnson. This conversation marked the beginning of our now over a decade-long collaboration into exploring links between Framework for Integration and ballroom dance technique. I am going to share a couple of these findings here.

The spiral arrangement of our musculature gives us the opportunity for a continuous, smooth movement across the floor. The opposing spirals give us the stability and support needed to perform complicated dance choreography with lightness and ease.

Let's start by demonstrating a typical standard dance position.

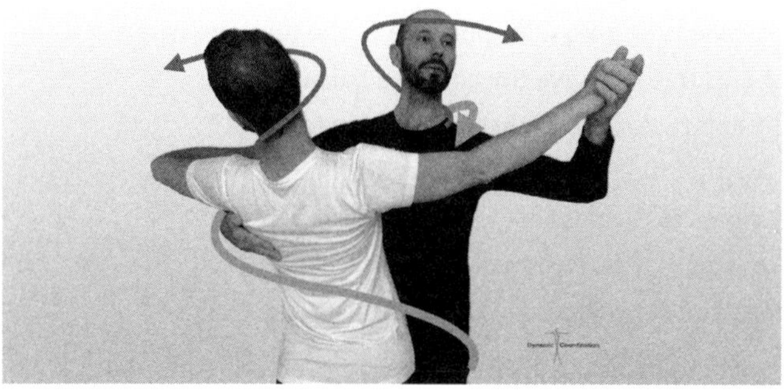

When connecting with a partner, both the leader and follower have gentle spirals to the right through their torsos (also through the legs, but we won't discuss it here). The head of each partner, however, does not follow that rightward spiral but opposes it by turning to the left. This opposition of spirals creates a wringing feeling, as in wringing the water out of a washcloth. This oppositional arrangement gives the body a natural sense of stability and support, without the need for stiffening and bracing.

You can also clearly see the same kind of opposition as we move to promenade position (where both partners face in the same direction).

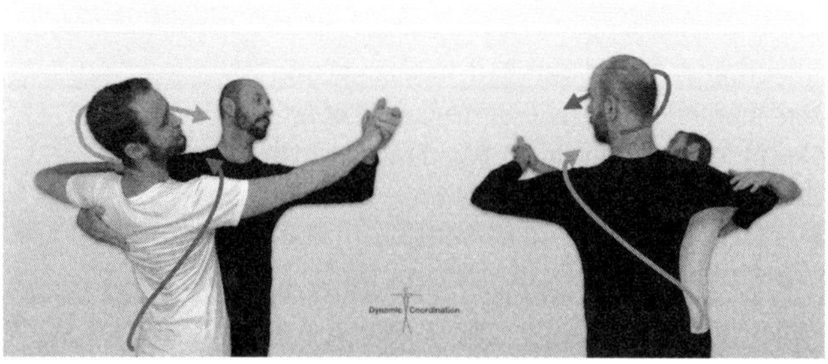

Here, the directions of spirals stay the same for the leader but change for the follower (body spirals to the left, head to the right).

This natural opposing of spirals gives ballroom dancing its characteristic continuity and smoothness in transitions from one rotation to the next. In competitive style, these opposing spirals are taken further, depending on the dancers' mobility. This opposition sometimes creates an illusion of an enormous shape, which is quite often mistaken by laypeople as leaning back. A closer look at highly skilled couples will reveal that it is in fact the opposition (the antagonistic actions) that creates the volume of the dancers' frame.

Spiral arrangement of human voluntary musculature is not limited to the torso and neck, but it also continues into the limbs. We will now explore how spirals in the arms help us achieve a stable, yet flexible dance hold.

First, let's revisit the concept of Primary and Secondary curves by performing the following exercise:

MOVEMENT EXPLORATION 15.1:
ARM ROTATIONS (SIMILAR TO MOVEMENT EXPLORATION 4.1)

While standing, drop the gaze toward the sternum, allowing the head and upper back to follow into Primary. Notice that when you don't interfere, the arms will start to rotate forward in the shoulders. Come back to standing position.

Now do the opposite: start looking up, allowing the head to follow and move the torso into Secondary. Notice that when doing this, the arms naturally rotate outward, toward what we call "anatomical position."

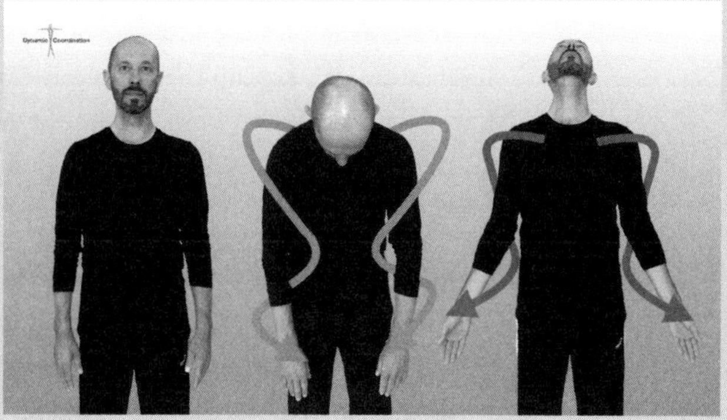

This simple exploration demonstrates that arms can also be moved toward Primary or Secondary. Moreover, the arms' movement will influence the torso accordingly.

Now, let's complicate things a bit. Open the arms to the side, about shoulder height, and ever so slightly engage the forward rotation in the shoulders toward Primary (don't allow the upper back to hunch forward). While maintaining the Primary in the shoulders, start to rotate in the forearms toward Secondary (supinate), thus feeling the opposing spirals through both arms. Now bend both arms toward a dance hold from the leader's perspective.

Now, let's do the opposite. Open the arms to the side again, at shoulder height, and engage the Secondary in the shoulders (outward rotation), this time allowing the torso to respond with slight Secondary engagement (typical of a follower in ballroom). While maintaining this engagement, rotate the forearms toward Primary

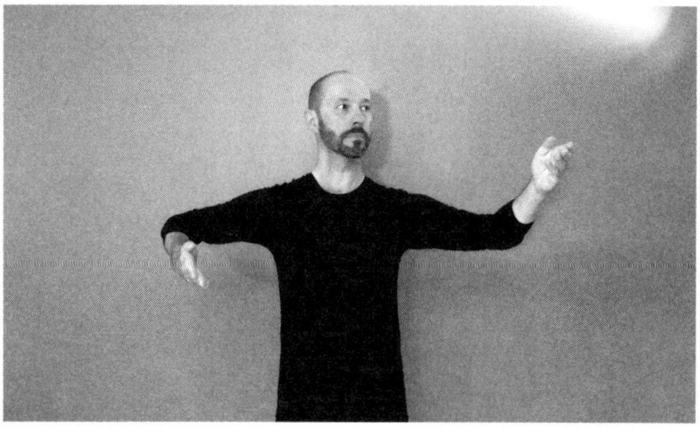

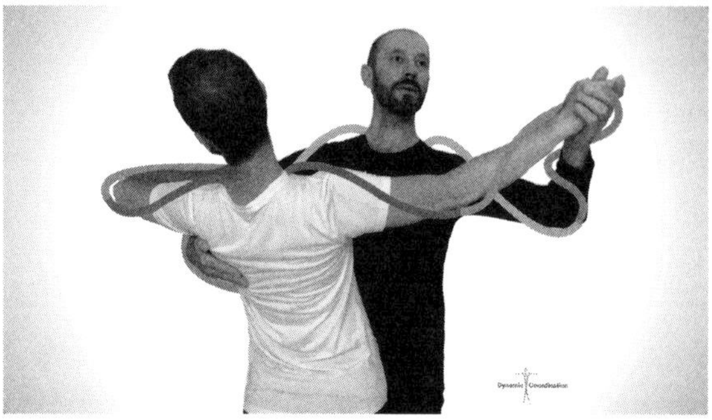

(pronate). Bend the elbows toward a dance hold from the follower's perspective.

Notice now how these two versions fit together to form a dance hold between two partners. This spiral arrangement allows for a natural tone in the frame without creating rigidity or a feeling of overpowering the partner. It also gives a sense of lift through the torso and the frame, giving a strong but flexible foundation for partner dancing.

These examples are just few of the many instances where Framework for Integration can explain the ballroom dance technique in clear, understandable terms without incorporating some overused ballroom jargon, which doesn't always describe the actions needed to be performed by the dancers. I use concepts of Framework for Integration in my daily ballroom dance lessons with great success.

Alex Tecza has been competing, performing, and teaching ballroom for over thirty years to students of all ages and abilities. Through his collaboration with Rebecca Nettl-Fiol on researching links between ballroom technique and Framework for Integration, Alex expanded his interests to Alexander Technique, developmental movement, Dart Procedures, and other somatic practices, and qualified as a teacher of the Alexander Technique in 2020. Since then, he has been researching applications of spirals in the teaching of ballroom dancing as well as in other forms of movement. (See dynamiccoordination.com for further information.)

Framework for Integration & Aerial Arts— "A Basic Invert"

Chandler Vaccaro

Many beginner pole-dancing students' first hurdle is a basic invert. The move is a prerequisite for most intermediate and advanced pole tricks, and it requires the strength and coordination to lift oneself off the floor. Luckily, my first introduction to basic inverts came not too long after my introduction to ball work and the Four Phases. Within the Framework, we explore the exchange of Engage and Reset between the Upper and Lower Triangles of the body. Rather than recruiting all Engagement for every activity, we learn how the Reset of some parts supports the overall movement of the whole.

After my pole teacher explained the initial concept of inverting, I watched several students' valiant attempts at the basic invert. I was still unconvinced the move would work until I began to recognize the ball work/Four Phases within the move. Gripping the pole and engaging through the Upper Triangle meant the Lower

Triangle was actually free to float up, or Reset, if I would only allow it. Excited to realize the Framework even had a place in my pole classes, I felt brave enough to explore.

As I set up my stance at the pole per the teacher's instructions, I thought through how this move would translate on the ball—as I engaged through my arms (the Upper Triangle), the *ball* would need to move forward (via the Reset of the Lower Triangle) to lift my hips parallel to my shoulders (or even higher!). I tightened my grip and pulled down on the pole, I felt the familiar sensation of being guided through the Four Phases on the ball—Primary Ball Forward (*Beach Chair*)—and whoosh! I simply floated in space, feeling amazed and in awe.

The resulting weightlessness from this integration led to a successful first attempt at the move, and many more styles of inverts to follow. Since beginning pole dancing, I've also taken up aerial silks and the Lyra (aerial hoop). While each apparatus has its own set of skills and tricks to master, they all incorporate the basic invert.

The beauty and utility of the Framework is that it provides a methodical, practical, and multi-step way to discover the Alexander Technique direction of "up" in more ways than one. As I've progressed into more advanced moves, using the Framework has allowed me to take the traditional AT directions into multiple planes and orientations—upside down and sideways, spinning around, and static. Whenever I'm feeling stuck in a move, or I have a sense I'm not moving as fluidly as I could be, the Framework becomes a diagnostic tool to unravel the hidden potential in each movement.

Departing from traditional AT methods (starting from the head/neck/back relationship), the Framework allows me to begin my analysis from any point in the body. For example, in a move called an allegra, your body is contorted around the pole in a backbend with arms reaching back behind you to touch one foot, while the other leg is extended into the air. Using the tools of both the Four Phases and the spirals, I can break down where the move is taking my body in space and use that intentionality to organize my movement. Maybe my gaze isn't following the line of movement that would allow my body to organize in space, or tension in my leg is contracting away from that line of movement. Aesthetically, I find a lack of flexibility can be somewhat overcome by moving the body with itself rather than against itself. When the body is working in concert, each move becomes more comfortable and fluid, to both the mover and the observer.

Several times throughout my aerial journey, I have been asked by other students, "What else do you do?" They tend to assume I am working out religiously in other ways outside of the studio to obtain the strength and coordination I'm often able to exhibit when learning new moves. Humbly and honestly, my main form of exercise over the last four years has been in the aerial dance studio. I'm not particularly interested in traditional workouts and have foregone many other activities to focus on aerial arts. While, of course, time put into any activity will increase one's comfort and ease with the activity, it's hard to imagine a similar progression without the knowledge of Alexander Technique and the tools of Framework for Integration. Studying both has dramatically altered my approach to all movement, whether that movement has been reaching for a cup of coffee, sitting to write for a book contribution, or flipping and flying through the air around a pole.

Video: A Basic Invert

Chandler Vaccaro grew up in a ballet studio but never really considered herself exceptionally coordinated or graceful until years of yoga, rock-climbing, and, ironically, sitting Zen meditation led her to the Alexander Technique. She holds a Bachelor of Science in Exercise Science and teacher certifications in both yoga and Pilates. Chandler considers learning and sharing the Alexander Technique her "PhD study" in movement studies. She teaches in Salt Lake City, enjoying AT in the air and on a pole when not teaching.

Chapter 16

Guest Contributions—Music Applications

Five musicians share their perspectives on working with the Framework principles in relation to conducting, singing, playing violin, teaching students to play stringed instruments, and playing harp.

Balancing Effort with Ease in Singing and Conducting

Jean Applonie

As a young singer and conductor with an overachiever mentality, I thought *doing* was the name of the game. And doing more could only be better. But I learned that some letting go was also required, which implied an ability to relax to some degree while singing and conducting. During my training, I gained a vague understanding of the need to work certain parts of my instrument while not working other parts, but I certainly was not taught any processes that would develop my skill and proficiency in balancing effort with ease during singing or conducting.

Hence, in my fifties, the concept of Reset was a happy revelation to me. I realized that I was not Resetting in my singing, in my conducting, in my workouts, even in my life. No wonder I had chronic headaches, backaches, and fatigue. I was never allowing pause for that brief moment of Reset between Engaged states. I somehow stayed in a state of fairly constant Engagement, feeling overly fatigued often. As a singer, I didn't know that I could allow each inhale to be a mini-Reset, briefly allowing tension to release and effort to ease. Instead, I experienced tension accumulating without relief. I was not using each new inhale to release minor tension built up during the singing of one breath/musical phrase. Imagine a song as a relay race, with each breath phrase as a leg of the race with a separate runner. Instead of the first runner winding down and resting after the baton handoff, imagine her continuing to run, even though the next runner has taken over (which could be seen as the next breath). Fatigue will set in quickly, and that initial runner will feel the need to work harder and harder to keep up the pace. Because of this accumulating tension, I would even use unnecessary effort to inhale.

To re-teach breath, I use the Alexander tool "Whispered Ah" (see reference in Chapter Eleven on Breathing) as a starting point for all my singers, simply allowing air to enter on its own, silkily and silently, not pulling it into the throat and lungs, and then exhaling on a Whispered Ah. The breath cycle of inhale and exhale is an ideal application of the Reset/Engage/Reset/Engage experience for a singer. I see the inhale as a Reset, while the exhale is Engaged. I relate a subtle Primary feeling in the spine to the inhale and a gentle Secondary feeling to the exhale. When I work with students, I allow space to explore this historic exercise nontraditionally, finding the option that works best for each individual. Some variations are: upright standing, upright sitting, hands supported on the back of a chair or on a table, hands resting on the seat of a chair in a four-legged position, and full body prone on a table with upper body resting on the wide end of a wedge pillow and the head propped on a stack of books at the forehead, jaw free to move into the Ah shape without running into the pillow. Every student has found at least one of these choices to be comfortable in practicing Whispered Ah. Quickly, they find they can release unnecessary tension in the larynx, throat, tongue, and jaw, as well as in the neck, shoulders, hips, and abdomen.

Weightlifting is another application I use for practicing Reset and Engage, for my own workouts and for giving Alexander students the feeling of Engage and Reset. I encourage the coordination of exhale with Engage when lifting the weight and an inhale with Reset when lowering the weight. Similar to my singing experience above, in my own weightlifting practice, I was not using the breath as a Reset to release building tension. Though I thought I was supporting goals of personal health and strength, I hated these workouts and ended them feeling exhausted. Now I am aware of the Secondary happening in my head/neck/back during a lift, which I do on an exhale. Then, I allow the inhale to release the effort in a Reset and my head/neck/back to spring back into a gentle Primary. Weightlifting is also a great way to practice using the Alexander principle of Whole Self. I encourage students to pause or inhibit just before lifting to imagine where their arms begin, at the inner clavicle notch in front and the vertebrae in back. Then I cue them to find their head, neck, back, and legs to all support the lift.

Another Framework concept that has transformed my coaching of singers in rehearsal is Primary and Secondary intentions. I now teach singers to identify their Primary or Secondary tendencies in standing and sitting positions. Many have a strong Secondary low back, both seated and standing. By releasing the hips to send the *ball* forward a bit they are much more comfortable at the end of a two-hour rehearsal. Those who have a tendency toward Primary in the upper body can be encouraged to lengthen the front body and/or look up a bit with their eyes, including an imaginary third eye, just below the notch between the clavicles. In coaching individual singers, I often find hips held in front of the shoulders or shoulders held in front of hips. By aligning the hips and shoulders, the singer naturally lengthens and feels less effort in being upright, and their ribcage's expansion is less impeded during the inhale.

Next, taking the Primary/Secondary concepts into spiraling, I discovered some valuable conducting applications. As the conductor gestures away from the center of the body on a beat one or three, the arm opens, turning slightly in a Secondary spiral and supinating. As the gesture returns inward toward the center of the body on a beat two or four, the arm spirals in Primary, pronating. I discovered that I was not allowing all the spiraling happening in my conducting arms to continue in my torso in a natural cycle of Engage/Reset/Engage/Reset as my arm swooped away from my body in a Secondary spiral and toward my body in a Primary spiral. When I allowed my ribs, even my hips to move with the spiraling arms and my weight to transfer to one leg, I could illustrate a more powerful legato line in my gesture, evoking a stronger, sustained tone from my singers. The full-body spiral also allowed me to scan the wide arc of my singers and make eye contact with every section. I found I could also spiral my torso in the opposite direction of my gesture, much like a string player's torso can spiral in the same direction as the bow or in the opposite direction to the bow. And, like in the weightlifting example above, employing the full body spiral is another means of practicing the AT principle of Whole Self.

Later, in teaching conducting gestures and patterns, I found that using Primary/pronating and Secondary/supinating spirals facilitates all the shifting angles of the palm, wrist, and forearm in one organic motion. Conducting is often taught as a two-dimensional, geometric pattern of angles executed by the palm, wrist, and forearm. This can result in a robotic piecing together of positions and parts rather than a natural, continuous flow of spiraling movement. Teaching my conducting students Primary/Secondary spirals was more successful overall and generated success more quickly than my previous methods of teaching angles, patterns, and body parts.

From the complex spiraling of arms and whole body to the simplicity of taking a single breath, I have found great use for the Framework concepts of Engage/Reset, Primary/Secondary intentions, and Primary/Secondary spirals. Informed by the natural functioning of the body (lungs, spine, and muscles), these processes enable me and my students to balance effort with ease in singing and conducting.

Jean Applonie has been a professional choral music conductor and teacher for thirty-eight years. She received her bachelor's and master's degrees from Brigham Young University, where she taught for twenty years, directing the BYU Women's Chorus and teaching music education. She enjoys dance as a hobby. She trained with Luc Vanier, Elizabeth Johnson, and Cathy Pollock in the charter group of graduates from the Salt Lake City Alexander Teacher Training course, certifying with the American Society for the Alexander Technique.

Framework for Integration Applications in Teaching String Instruments: When in Doubt, Up and Out!

Jenna Baumgart

One would think that musicians would understand that movement is integral to playing their instruments, but this isn't necessarily so. We must move to produce sound, whether internal (vocal) or external (with an instrument or other noise maker). However, the false sensory aspect of movement affects musicians to the degree that pain while playing is prevalent. Also, in my own experience, I have found that the sound produced becomes more open and free if the musician works under less tension and is less static.

I have implemented spirals with my high school orchestras and found that the addition of directed movement, while foreign at the beginning, makes my groups sound and feel better. Like any new concept, some students are hesitant to buy in, but if they pay attention, they hear the difference and allow movement to become part of their performance.

Spirals have a natural place in a musician's movement. As a string player, the bow is one place to think about a spiral. The inward spiral should be apparent if we think about strength and speed while watching someone throw a punch (in slow motion). Try it. If you attempt to punch straight forward in the sagittal plane, how much force is behind that? Versus allowing the arm to spiral, bringing the motion of the punch where it naturally wants to go, which is a bit inward, how much more force do you feel behind this, and likely with less effort?

I adjust bowing terminology to "up and out" vs. "up and down." The idea of down pulls our bodies in that direction, and is the direction of the bow actually "down"? Moving the bow in a typical "up and out" fashion, we can imagine the spiral in the arm, even exaggerate it as we move. This spiral is natural from the wrist and fingers to forearm to the upper arm.

Bowing a string instrument has little difference from throwing the punch; the plane, direction, and intent behind the motion are the difference. The natural weight and strength behind the spiral allow for better contact with the string, and better sound production, allowing the string to spin (spiral), resulting in more unrestrained sound and better tone production.

To broaden this, I take the spiral movement to the entire body, both seated and standing. We start simply by finding our sitz bones by rocking back and forward and side to side on them. Sometimes I make the students sit on their hands to find the bones as they move. Often they find that they are not sitting on them but are far in front or, more usually, behind them.

From here, we talk about spirals in general, things like DNA as the basic building block of our bodies, and how muscles wrap around, so why wouldn't the rest of us spiral? Sometimes this involves the overweight, fifty-plus-year-old teacher demonstrating how to spiral to the ground and spiral up. This demonstration usually elicits giggles, but more often, they are amazed that I can get down and up more easily than most of them.

Then we spiral in the chair without our instruments. Make sure that feet can reach the floor and we have room to move without hitting each other. I reiterate that they should feel their sitz bones and that their weight should end up there and transfer as they spiral side to side.

It is here that one can see patterns and habits. Are their heads turning with their body? Are arms free or firm? Do the legs give up weight as they shift from one side to the other? Admittedly, several students will be uncomfortable with moving or cannot do it because of holding patterns that have long been ingrained as a habit. Here, I use pedagogical touch if the student permits, directing their head, arms, or legs to release and either lead or follow the movement.

Then, we add their instrument (without the bow) and continue the exploration of spirals with their instrument in hand. For cellists, this becomes an interesting prospect, and I offer two ways; they can either keep their endpin out and turn the instrument with them or pull the endpin in and sit baroque style with the instrument only between their knees and spiral with it there. Note that baroque style may cause more holding if a student is less experienced or unfamiliar with the technique. In those instances, it may not be the best idea. Bass players usually have little difficulty with this once they figure out how to shift weight and balance on both feet.

Then we put the bow in hand and do something simple, like a one-octave scale. The caveat is that tone and pitch are not the focus. The focus is *movement*! Allow them to make pitch and fingering errors. Let them be OK with mistakes. No one cares. There is always the in-between option to bow without the bow, just making the motion in the arm and continuing to focus more on the spiral itself. Once using the bow, we move the bow in the same direction we are spiraling, keeping in mind "up and out"; otherwise, "down" is the direction the body will go!

Often I find that this is enough for several weeks of work. Putting an unfamiliar skill with one that, for many string students, is almost automatic throws them for the proverbial loop. Again, pedagogical touch for direction is helpful. There is no way to stay on the podium and direct this activity well. Also, be cognizant of students who may be developmentally behind or your special needs students; allow them to do what they can without pressure or being put on the spot.

From here, we will spiral opposite the bow direction, use different scales, and have the violin and viola players walk around the cellists/bassists, having the low string players spiral in the direction the upper strings are walking.

Of course, the most challenging thing is putting this into practice in an actual piece of music. That said, I doubt you want your group to make the audience seasick, so a happy medium must be reached.

Reminders of movement are often enough once you have put the practice into place. The idea of moving is helpful internally and usually allows the body to free itself in areas where tension is being held, unknown to the musician. Pointing this out as students learn the art of moving again is revelatory for many of them.

Video: Application for Musicians—When in Doubt, Up and Out

Jenna Baumgart is a violinist and public school music educator in Utah. She holds a bachelor's and a master's degree in Music Education from Utah State University and the University of Utah, respectively. Her tension-induced injuries led her to the AT and to become an AT teacher. Subsequently, AT and the Framework have become an integral part of her teaching in helping young musicians learn to become aware of their habits and to play tension free.

Coordination Underlying Musical Intention at the Harp: Using the Framework to Observe Ourselves in Activity

Claire Happel Ashe

At eighteen, I wanted nothing more than to be immersed in modern dance and harp performance. I imagined moving to a vibrant city, far from my small hometown in Illinois, where I could begin a fascinating and hip life in the arts. However, as I researched schools, I discovered that the University of Illinois Urbana-Champaign, my state's flagship institution, offered standout programs in both fields. Despite my initial reluctance to stay nearby, those programs became a reason to do so. My decision to attend U of I proved to be a particularly serendipitous one because two faculty were working out concepts at that very moment that became a defining part of my life's work and integrated my two fields of harp and movement. Those two individuals were Becky and Luc, and their ideas are the most potent system for understanding movement and developing skill that I have encountered, a system that is now called Framework for Integration.

During my classes with Becky and Luc, I had several transformative experiences that resonated so fundamentally with everything I did that I could not help but look for applications everywhere. The first insight came about when I experienced the spiral musculature. By looking over my shoulder, which engaged the spiral, I experienced a release in my lower back, increased freedom in my legs, and the ability to be more grounded on my standing leg. This pattern improved my jumps, "alignment," and overall sense of connection in dance classes. The second insight occurred when Luc asked me to direct my intention outward, reaching toward an "imaginary cookie," which incited a strong Secondary throughout my entire being. It made it clear that postural and movement patterns stem from intention and are deeply a part of our system. Those insights compelled me to explore how the work applied to other areas of life and, most important, the harp. I began examining how intention and the spiral musculature bring about freedom, strength, and virtuosity in harp performance.

Below are various applications of the Framework for harpists. The applications are also applicable to skills beyond harp performance that involve fine motor movement or musical intention.

1. Simple Model
   - The action of being seated behind the harp is a more Primary use of the limbs in general (bending, flexing affinity of the limbs in front of the spine).
   - Closing the fingers is a Primary action (bending, softening, curling in, flexing affinities); reaching toward the strings is a Secondary action (extending, going out into the world affinities).
   - The use of the thumbs is a more Primary action (push affinity), and use of the opposing fingers is a more Secondary action (pull affinity). The relationship of the push and pull of the thumb and fingers is facilitated by the elbows and hips in opposition. Find these affinities by pushing and pulling a chair or playing the harp while seated on the ball.

Video: Application for Musicians: Coordination Underlying Musical Intention at the Harp, Part 1

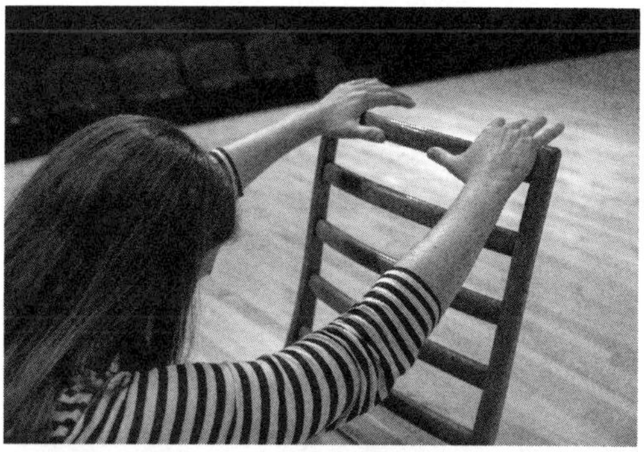

Hands on the back of the chair pushing (*Primary ball back*)

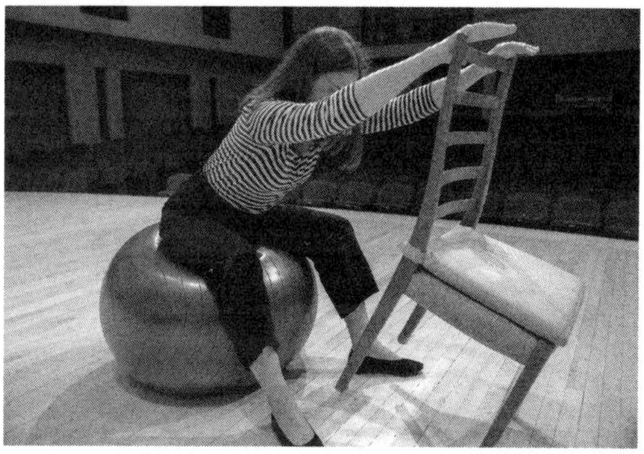

Hands on the back of the chair pushing (*Primary ball back*)

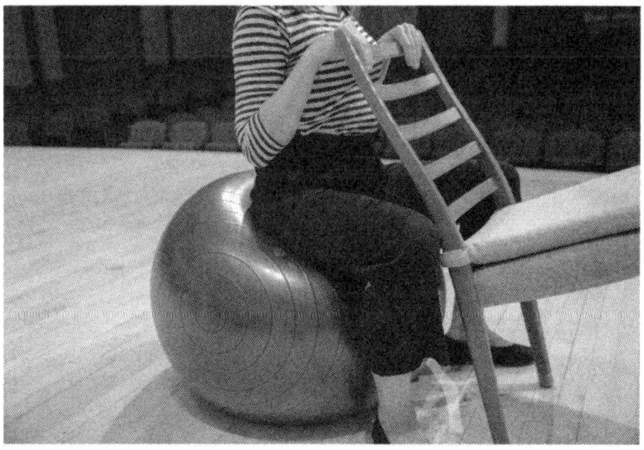

Hands on the back of the chair pulling (*Secondary ball forward*)

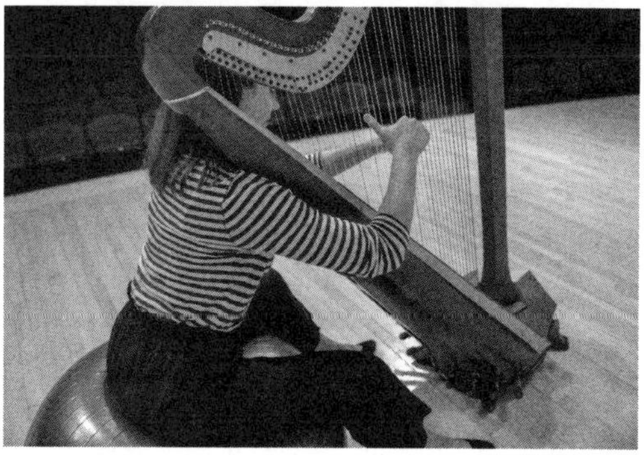

Thumbs on the harp (*Secondary* ball back)

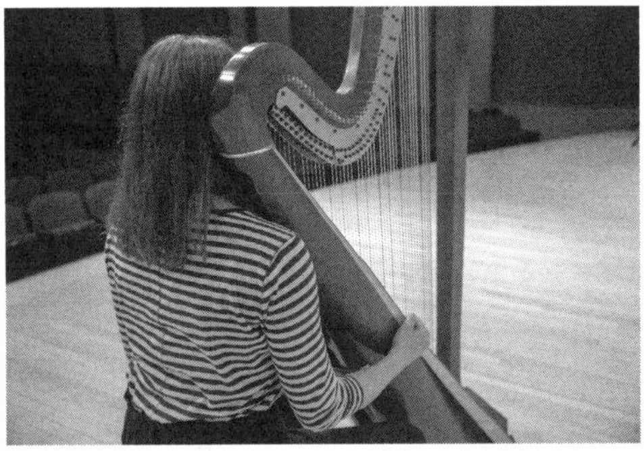

Right shoulder supporting the harp in spiral to the left

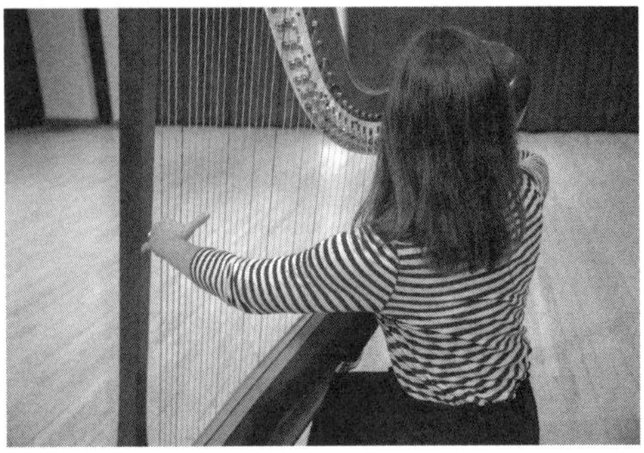

Left hand reaching into the bass register in spiral to the right

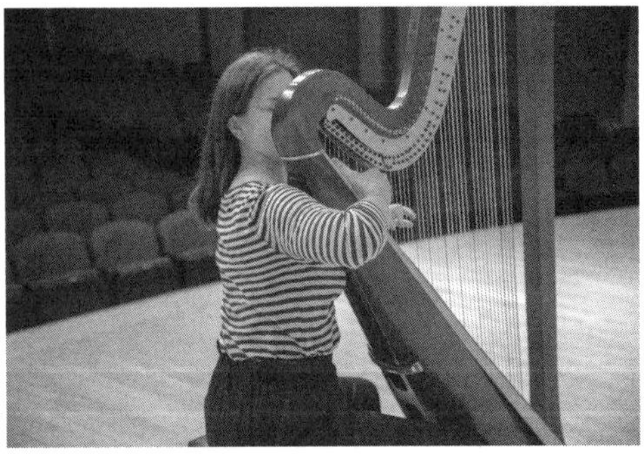

Both hands in the upper register in spiral to the right

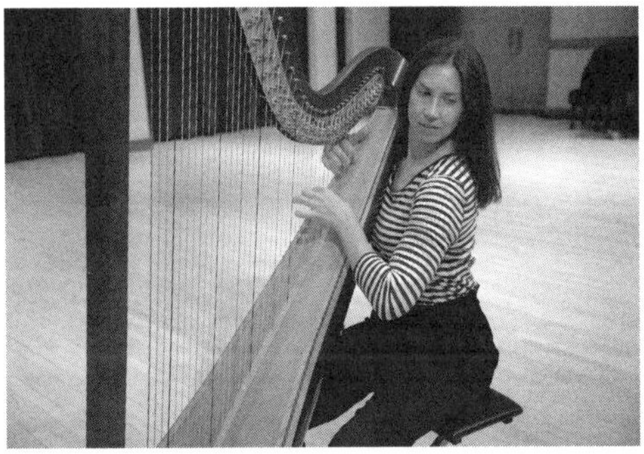

Interlocking spiral: shoulders to the right and head to the left

2. Complex Model

- Supporting the harp on the right shoulder leads to a Primary action of the right shoulder to bear the weight of the harp, spiraling the torso to the left.

In the complex model, we can see the many ways that spirals support us at the harp.

Video: Application for Musicians: Coordination Underlying Musical Intention at the Harp, Part 2

- The use of the right hand in the treble register and the left hand in the bass leads to a spiral of shoulders to the right.

Video: Application for Musicians: Coordination Underlying Musical Intention at the Harp, Part 3

- The head looking at the conductor or music to the left, in opposition to the shoulders spiraled to the right, is an interlocking spiral. Looking at the upper strings is a single spiral in the direction of shoulders to the right.

Video: Application for Musicians: Coordination Underlying Musical Intention at the Harp, Part 4

- Lifting a foot to move to various pedals necessitates a spiral in the whole back to free up the leg in Primary, which engages the other foot into the floor in Secondary.

Video: Application for Musicians: Coordination Underlying Musical Intention at the Harp, Part 5

- The use of the legs to engage the pedals is a spiraled action of pronation to press it out and release it up, and supination to pull it in and push it down.

Video: Application for Musicians: Coordination Underlying Musical Intention at the Harp, Part 6

- The Secondary and Primary motion of opening and closing to play a chord at the harp has an underlying double spiral balanced between pronation and supination that supports the opening and closing motion. This mirrors the underlying double spiral that supports the head looking up and down.
- Typically (but not always), the spiral of pronation supports plucking toward the thumb, and the spiral of supination supports plucking away from the thumb. The spiraled action of supination and pronation in the arms happens in coordination with the fingers' reaching (Secondary) and grasping (Primary).
- Suggested hand positions at the harp can be seen through the lens of interlocking spirals in the arms. The Salzedo method seems to use a pronating upper arm against a supinating lower arm, while the Grandjany method seems to use a supinating upper arm against a pronating lower arm.

Video: Application for Musicians: Coordination Underlying Musical Intention at the Harp, Part 7

Video: Application for Musicians: Coordination Underlying Musical Intention at the Harp, Part 8

- The interlocking spiral creates a strong coil to pluck the strings that then releases in the opposite spiral after closing. The interlocking spiral of the arm and its use in a pull (Secondary) or push (Primary) will have an effect on the Upper and Lower Triangles of the torso.

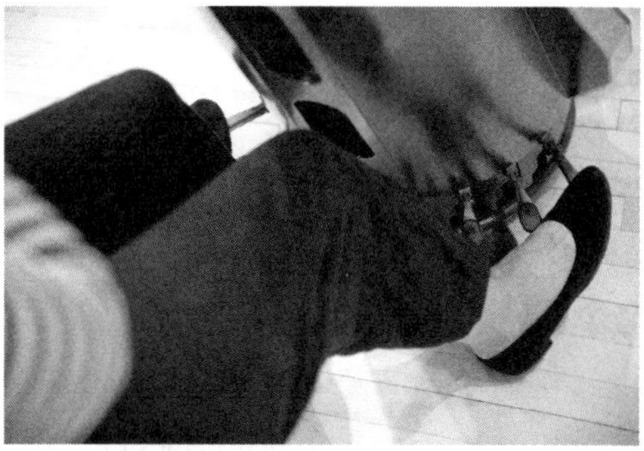

Pronating the feet to release the pedals upward

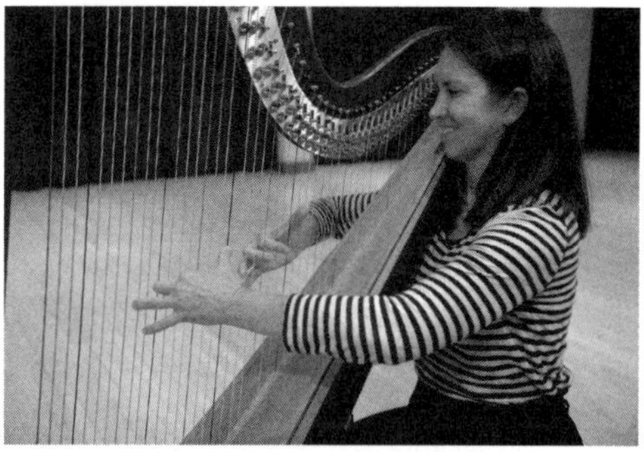

Salzedo hand position before plucking

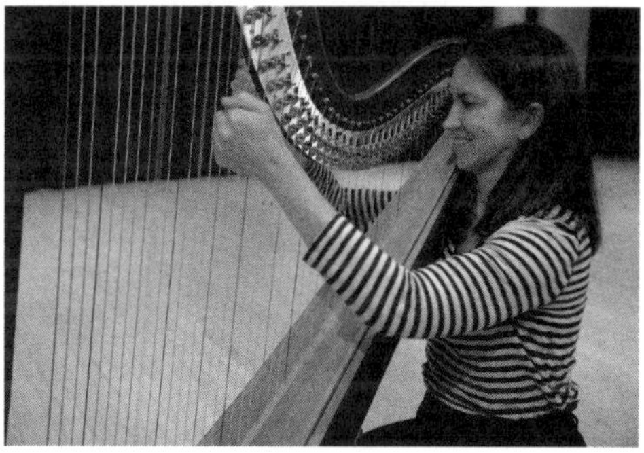

Salzedo hand position after plucking

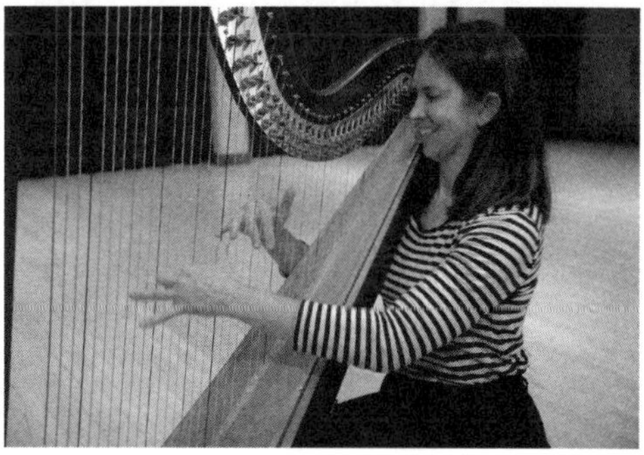

Grandjany hand position before plucking

3. Integrated Model

   - The Four Phases can be applied to playing chords: plucking as a Primary Engagement; the bounce out of palms as a Secondary Reset; reaching to the strings as a Secondary Engagement; and folding the fingers onto strings as a Primary Reset. There are various responses to these phases throughout the whole body that can be observed to notice interference and holding.

In musical motion downward and upward, Engagements and Resets between the thumb and opposing fingers can create strong/weak rhythmic cycles. A pronated engagement (pull) of the opposing finger(s) creates a rhythmically strong note leading to a supinated Reset in the thumb that is rhythmically weak. Conversely, a supinated engagement (push) of the thumb creates a rhythmically strong note that leads to a pronated Reset in the opposing finger(s) that is rhythmically weak. Engaged arm spirals and their Reset in the opposite spiral can be experienced while seated on the ball and pulling/pushing an object or the strings at the harp.

Video: Application for Musicians: Coordination Underlying Musical Intention at the Harp, Part 9

Video: Application for Musicians: Coordination Underlying Musical Intention at the Harp, Part 10

When the hands are not in unison, Engagements to bring out various notes of the melody also create spirals in the torso that Reset. For example, in an arpeggio downward, starting with the right hand while emphasizing the first note, the engaged push of the right thumb will spiral the torso to the left and then Reset through the rest of the fingers. In an arpeggio upward, beginning with the left hand and emphasizing the lowest note, the engaged pull of the left-hand fourth

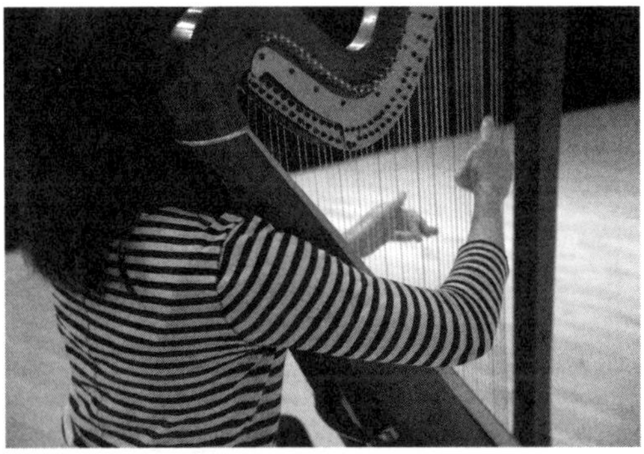

Push of the right thumb in downward arpeggio, spiraling the shoulders to the left

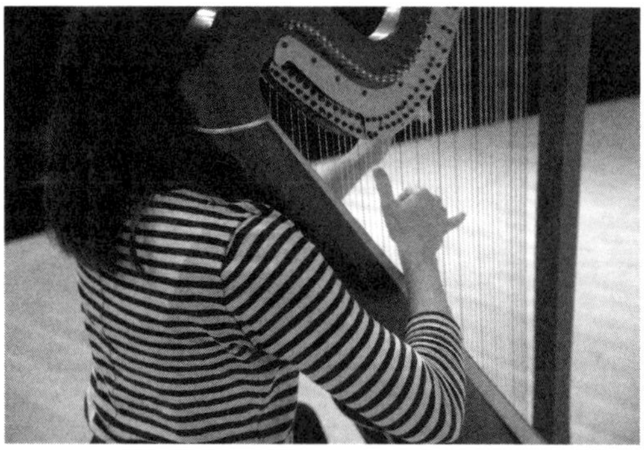

Reset of the shoulders to the right

finger will spiral the torso to the right and Reset through the rest of the fingers upward.

Video: Application for Musicians: Coordination Underlying Musical Intention at the Harp, Part 11

The second example of the Integrated Model mentioned above highlights the significance of rhythmic intention within the Integrated Model of the Framework. During my study of Baroque performance practice with historical harpist Cheryl Ann Fulton, I found that her approach to paired fingerings, known as the "good" and "bad" notes of Baroque performance practice, was an excellent example of rhythmic intention leading to Engagements and Resets. In her technique called the "wave," as in the second example above, she uses pronation of the fingers and supination of the thumb to create rhythmic cycles of engaged, rhythmically strong articulations leading to Reset, rhythmically weak articulations.

The Framework provides a comprehensive perspective to examine diverse individual approaches to the harp, such as those of Cheryl Ann Fulton, by looking at the entire pattern of an action and its outcome. This broader perspective allows for greater choice, because isolated or competing instructions within harp methods can be analyzed within a larger context. Performers can then choose patterns based on their musical needs and notice how well the patterns they are using accomplish their musical intentions. Individualized instructions on position become opportunities to understand the underlying pattern used, as seen in the Complex Model applied to the Salzedo and Grandjany harp methods above. Perhaps the two harpists' differing musical intentions for sound, rhythm, and phrasing led to the physical patterns they advocated.

During my undergraduate years, Luc asked me to present to my fellow dance classmates about the connections I discovered at the harp. Despite their lack of musical training, they still found the ideas engaging because underlying aspects of intention, dynamic spirals, balance, and timing are fundamental to all skills. More than twenty years later, the ideas in the Framework continue to evolve and remain as resonant, exciting, and potent as ever. I hope they are as fascinating to you as they were and still are to me.

Video: Application for Musicians: Coordination Underlying Musical Intention at the Harp—Synthesis Plus Performance

Note: All photos and videos by Philip Weiss, WIU School of Music

Claire Happel Ashe is a harpist and teacher with a background in dance. As a harpist, she frequently performs with ensembles throughout the Midwest, including the Saint Louis Symphony Orchestra, Newberry Consort, and her own chamber ensemble, River Town Duo. She holds degrees in music from Yale University (M.M./A.D.) and the University of Illinois (B.M./D.M.A.), where she also received her B.F.A. in Dance and completed her doctoral thesis on the application of the Alexander Technique, Dart Procedures, and Framework for Integration to the harp.

A Violinist's Perspective: Four Movement Explorations

Laurie Shawger

Most of my career has been spent performing in a symphony orchestra, teaching young violinists, and occasionally performing chamber music or solos, a typical mix for a classical violinist. I have performed everywhere music goes, from barns (yes, plural), street corners, and sports stadiums to Carnegie Hall. My formal violin studies and conservatory training occurred in an era when warm up meant rinsing your hands in hot water, the sole focus of technique was the hands, and the body as a whole was largely ignored.

As the years passed, I found myself increasingly strained to meet the demands of a performing career and life in general. The popular image of musicians leading glamorous lives filled with high-profile concerts and elegant receptions in storied venues belies the reality of hours of disciplined practice, strenuous concert schedules, and the vagaries of performing situations. Professional musicians work in a culture that customarily normalizes and minimizes physical issues. Yet, the cost of disregarding the body is high.

I have benefited tremendously from using the Framework to better understand my movement habits and increase my options in managing myself, especially with the violin. The advantage of using a theory is that it is not clouded by my habits and preferences and therefore is useful to tease apart and test my movement beliefs and assumptions.

The explorations below outline a sequential progression of movement experiments. The text of each exploration provides a setup, instructions, and comments. Alexander Technique principles are integral to my practice but have not been restated in the instructions. Videos accompanying the explorations are provided to model the exploratory process, not an ideal result. Each video captures what was going on in the moment of negotiating habits while carrying out a movement intention. The learning from these explorations will emerge from your own experience and self-observation. I encourage you to realistically gauge your own balance and comfort level and move within that scope. Reminder pauses are indicated initially but are discontinued as the explorations progress. It is up to you to take time and thoughtfully pace yourself.

MOVEMENT EXPLORATION 16.1: WEIGHT TRANSFER, SIMPLE SPIRAL, COUNTER SPIRAL

Setup: Materials needed are four small balls. Consider the balls' softness and positioning for maximum comfort and feedback during this exploration. Stand upright, balanced with your weight evenly shared on both feet. Underneath each of your upper arms, place a ball against the side of your ribcage. In each hand, gently hold a ball resting against your thigh.

1. Take a moment to stand quietly and sense your breathing through feedback from the balls.
2. Facing forward, shift your weight onto your right leg, pause, and then come back to center with your weight balanced evenly on both feet. Pause.
3. Shift the weight onto your left leg. Pause and then move back to center.
4. Next, begin to look toward the right, allowing your head to turn to the right as you shift your weight onto your right leg. Pause. Notice if you allowed a Reset, then return to center, facing forward.
5. Repeat on the left side.
6. Next, while beginning to look toward the right and allowing your head to turn toward the right, shift your weight to the left leg. Pause, then move back to center.
7. Repeat on the other side.

Video: Weight Transfer, Simple Spiral, Counter Spiral

Comments: After you have moved through the exploration, go back and repeat steps 1 and 2. This time as you shift weight to the right, observe the connectivity engaged to support uprightness and consciously invite what is not needed to Reset. Do likewise as you shift weight toward the left.

Throughout steps 1–6, what did you notice about the small balls? Video yourself and take a look.

Did you allow the balls to roll? Did the balls on one side roll more than those on the other side? Comparing what you felt to what you saw in your video, were there any surprises?

It is normal to feel more comfortable turning to one side than to the other. Dart wrote, "any habitually asymmetrical adjustment of the body, either during states of mental anxiety that suppress respirational rhythm or during occupations or exercise, results in postural torsion of the head, vertebral column and trunk, as a whole, towards the right or towards the left (whichever is the more commonly used side)" (1996, 71).

MOVEMENT EXPLORATION 16.2:
WEIGHT TRANSFER WITH THE VIOLIN

Setup: Stand in a balanced, upright stance with your weight shared evenly on both feet, the instrument in playing position, and the bow held in your right hand, resting at your side. Remember to take your time and pause as needed.

1. Face forward and place the middle of the bow on one string. Without drawing the bow, shift your weight toward one foot, pause, then shift your weight toward the other foot. Repeat a couple of times. Are you allowing Resets to occur in relationship to the weight transfer?
2. Next, experiment with using your bow: On the down bow, shift weight to the right and on the up bow, shift weight to the left. Repeat a few times.

3. Then, try shifting weight in the direction opposite to the bow change. On the down bow, shift weight to the left and on the up bow, shift weight to the right. Repeat a few times.
4. The movement may organically extend into a more expansive spiral. Try changing the bow direction randomly as you wish, not aligned with the weight transfer.

Video: Weight Transfer with the Violin

Comments: Comparing the patterns in steps 2 and 3 above, which combination of weight transfer and bow direction feels more familiar?

In *The Teaching of Action in String Playing: Developmental and Remedial Techniques,* Rolland emphasized the function of weight transfer in playing string instruments to free up the body. Rolland used the term "unilateral movement" to describe when the bow and the weight transfer move in the same direction, as in step 2 above. He used the term "bi-lateral movement" to describe the bow and the weight transfer moving in contrary directions, as in step 3 above (Rolland 2007, 33–34).

Exploring spirals through the Framework lens has helped me develop an embodied understanding of the asymmetrical movements involved with playing the violin and the habits that I have intentionally or unintentionally cultivated.

MOVEMENT EXPLORATION 16.3: CIRCLES

Setup: Materials needed are a chair and your instrument.

Sit balanced and upright, approximately halfway toward the front edge of the chair, with both of your feet on the floor, the instrument in playing position, and the bow hand resting on your thigh.

1. Begin by looking toward one side as you allow your weight to shift to that side.
2. Continue looking outward at normal eye level and sweep your gaze around toward the front, as the torso inclines slightly toward the direction you are looking. The violin is carried along as the shoulders adapt to the circular movement. Allow the relationship between the head, the violin, and the torso to change responsively to the movement.
3. Continue sweeping your gaze around to the opposite side, then look down to your shoulder and across your chest as your back retreats slightly and your weight shifts.
4. Repeat the circle in the same direction. Pay attention to the connection between head and pelvis, as evidenced by the weight transfers. What else did you notice?
5. Repeat the movement, circling in the opposite direction. What did you observe?
6. Next, lightly play with the left fingers on the fingerboard as you again lead with your gaze to circle in the original direction. Pause, then repeat the circle in the opposite direction.
7. Stop the left-hand fingering and instead, begin bowing on an open string. Repeat the circles as described above.

Video: Circles

Comments: Sound quality is a useful source of information about general physical use in relation to the violin. Did you hear moments when the contact between the bow and the string changed? Did you observe any physical clues in the video that correlated with changes in the sound quality? Video yourself and watch for Engagements and Resets. On the playback, if your attention was on the upper body, watch again, observing your body as a whole. What was happening with the pelvis, legs, and feet?

MOVEMENT EXPLORATION 16.4: FIGURE EIGHT WITH THE VIOLIN

The figure eight is a fusion of the weight transfers and spirals/circles from the preceding explorations.

Figure 16.1 and 16.2 show the only two possible movement pathways for this continuous loop. The instructions below provide one option to initiate each movement pathway.

Setup: Stand and hold the violin in playing position without the bow.

Hint: In the figure eight, the shoulders and arms participate in the spiral connection that extends through the whole body. The relationship between the head, the violin, and the torso is not static; it continually adapts as the movement proceeds. Pay attention to Engagements and allow Resets.

Video: Figure Eight with the Violin

Figure 16.1 Movement Pathway

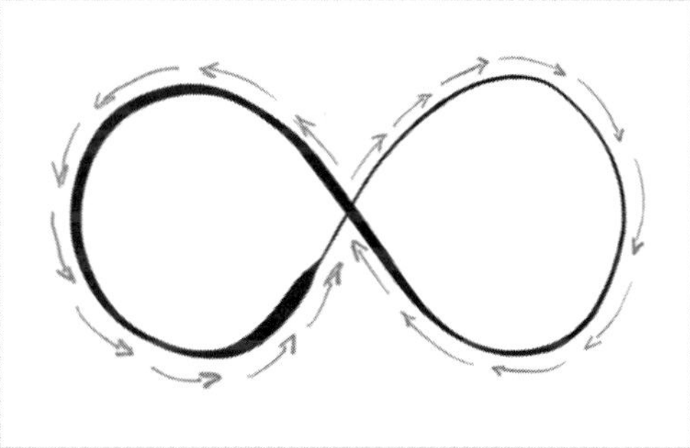

Figure 16.1

1. Look outward in front of you, then begin to circle your gaze to the right, let your head turn, allow your shoulders to spiral to the right, and let your weight shift to the right. The violin is carried along in the spiral.
2. Next, look down toward your right shoulder, let your back retreat slightly as your downward gaze passes across the front midline of your torso, and slowly raise your gaze up to look outward, slightly to the left of center front.
3. As you sweep your gaze around to the left, turn your head to the left, allow your left shoulder to spiral to the left, carrying the violin along with it, and allow your weight to shift to the left side.
4. Slowly drop your gaze down toward your left shoulder. Let your back retreat slightly as you bring your gaze past the midline of your torso, then begin to look up, finishing with your gaze directed forward at normal eye level.
5. Repeat steps 1–4 to repeat the same movement pathway.

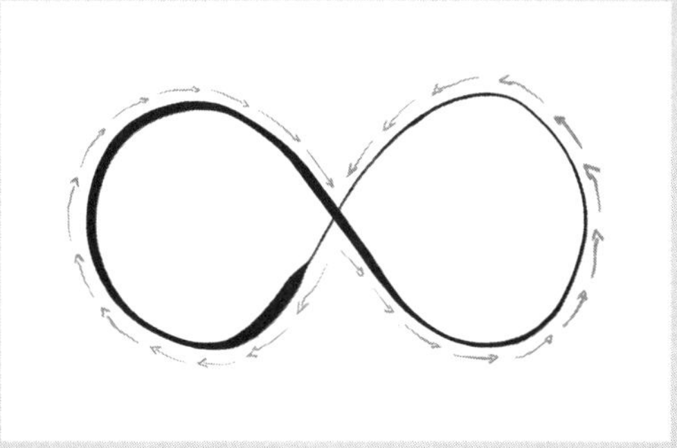

Figure 16.2

Figure 16.2 Movement Pathway

1. Looking downward toward the right shoulder, allow your weight to shift to the right as your shoulders participate in the spiral, carrying the violin along. Lift your gaze up and look outward as you sweep your gaze away from your right shoulder, leading your torso in an arc toward the left.
2. Just before your gaze has reached directly in front of you, look downward and let your back retreat slightly.
3. Let your downward gaze pass your midline toward the left. Turn your head toward your left shoulder, allowing your shoulders to participate in the spiral, carrying the violin along, as your weight shifts to the left.
4. Slowly bring your gaze up and direct it away from your left shoulder, turning your head to the right to lead your torso in an arc. The violin is carried along with the spiral.
5. Just before your gaze reaches center front, drop your gaze, and draw your downward gaze back to your chest as your back retreats slightly. Pass your gaze across the midline of your torso and then direct it toward your right shoulder as you turn your head to the right. The violin is carried along with the spiraling movement of the shoulders.
6. Repeat steps 1–5 to continue the same movement pathway.

Comments: The movement pattern I have conceptualized as a figure eight originally evolved in a lesson with Luc working with me and the violin. Exploring the habit-defying symmetry of the figure eight has been pivotal in building my experiential understanding of what is possible beyond my habitual movement patterns with and without the violin.

This exploration is challenging. Please be respectful of yourself and give yourself permission to take it easy, take a break, or try it on another day.

Using the Framework in Practice

This video is a demonstration of how I use the Framework in practicing the violin. The practice music is from the *Variations on a Gavotte by Corelli* by Henri Vieuxtemps. The video is not a performance and is not intended to represent ideals in technique, musicality, or any other facet of violin playing.

Video: Using the Framework in Practice—A Video of the Process

Conclusion

In this set of explorations, I have encouraged the reader to experience the organization of spiral connection through the whole body in relation to the violin. This approach has been important for my growth and learning. However, I recognize that there are many ways to carry out a movement intention. Mizrahi stated, "there exist multiple pathways for the performance of a given motor task such that a given central command may be executed in different ways and, conversely, the same end result can be triggered from different trigger commands. . . ." (2020, 5).

In my experience, when connectivity through the body is adaptively supporting movement through Engagements and Resets, my movement choices increase. In a given moment, options such as orienting aurally, or leading with an arm, hand, shoulder, or hip, may be available and well suited for initiating and supporting the intended movement. Applying the Framework to my experiential learning has helped me expand my available options in relation to the violin, a key factor for healthy activity and career longevity.

In terms of health and wellness, I have benefited tremendously from having a lens for experimentation outside of my habitual tendencies, while acknowledging and honoring the constraints that are present for me. Each person has their own unique situation and their personal path toward growth. Framework for Integration has continued to be a valuable tool for me to understand my movement tendencies, identify where interferences are occurring, and expand what is possible for me in a gentle, nonthreatening way.

Laurie Shawger, violinist, retired in 2023 after a thirty-four-year career in the Milwaukee Symphony Orchestra. She is an AmSAT certified Alexander Technique teacher. She taught violin for thirty-five years, including ten years on the faculty of the Wisconsin Conservatory of Music. Laurie earned Bachelor and Master of Music degrees at the Juilliard School. In 2022, she graduated from Mount Mary University with an M.S. in Clinical Mental Health Counseling and is in private practice. Her enduring interest is in the health and well-being of musicians.

Chapter 17

Guest Contributions—Mindful Movement Applications

The following contributions look at ways to think about the Framework in somatic practices including yoga, Tai-Chi Chuan, and meditation.

Yoga: Simple, Complex, and Integrated Model Applications in Foundational Asanas

Elizabeth Johnson

As a contemporary dancer, I was peripherally aware that many of the movements I practiced had yogic influences, especially some of the more "traditional" forms like Graham technique. In the late 1990s, my initial introduction to yoga was through fitness culture—the gym was a place where I could entrust my three young children to hourly daycare so I could have a few moments to take a class. I stumbled into teaching yoga in these same fitness contexts, my new practice and dance background as my only qualifications. Thanks to knowledgeable professors and peers, in graduate school I went on to deepen my personal practice and, over a decade later, became certified under the tutelage of an expert practitioner. I credit yoga practice as the place where I discovered and began paying attention to the rhythms and awareness of my breath. From those early years on, yoga asanas and practices have been threaded through my dance teaching and dance making.

Yoga in the United States is no stranger to colonial, Western tendencies to decontextualize, extract, and appropriate. Sacred spiritual origins and histories often are erased, with the asanas used as means to ends, especially goals for accomplishing feats of extreme flexibility. In the yoga classes I take and teach, I watch all different ages, genders, and kinds of bodies bearing burdens of internal and external pressures to push physical limits that are often questionable if not harmful. Yoga teachers generally recognize the lack of coordination and postural collapse in twenty-first-century bodies and strive to lift their students out of the concave torsos and tight hips engendered by desk and computer work, commutes in cars, and hunching over cell phones. From a Framework point of view, in the Simple Model, this would be recognizing the contracture of chronic Primary patterning. To address this observation, I often hear instructions to "pull shoulder blades back and down," "open and send the heart forward," and generally lengthen and spread the front of the body—an encouragement to extend more into an overall Secondary intent.

The beautiful thing about yoga sequences and asanas is, in the Simple Model, they naturally alternate between Primary and Secondary in the sagittal and vertical planes. A great example of this in standing would be reaching to the sky with arms overhead (*Urdhva Hastasana*), a fully extended Secondary reach, to fold forward (*Uttanasana*), a deep Primary rounding. Adding *ball* directions to this example can be helpful: Reaching up to the sky is *Seagulls* phase, with the *ball* going forward, and folding over is *Sandals* phase, sending the *ball* back.

Going through a simple cat (*Marjaryasana*) and cow (*Bitilasana*) sequence arching and rounding the spine on all fours, you can layer the recognition of Primary, Secondary, and the *ball* direction while also integrating an awareness of the arms to reveal the complex patterning of the Upper and Lower Triangles. In the push of the hands away from the mat in the rounded-back cat, the Upper is engaged with the Lower more released (feel how your arms can bear your weight and the knees can wiggle). If you pull to your hands, wrists, and elbows in the arched cow, shifting your weight slightly back to the lower body, the Lower is engaged (and the elbows can wiggle even mid-pull). These patterns appear over and over again in other asanas that build on the foundations of cat and cow. Cat patterning underlies the Primary push that facilitates and sustains downward-facing dog (*Adho Mukha Svanasana*) and inversions like headstand (*Sirsasana*). Cow patterns underlie the pull that facilitates and sustains cobra (*Bhujangasana*) and upward-facing dog (*Urdhva Mukha Svanasana*).

I find the Simple Model and the Integrated Model's Four Phases on the ball clarifying and fun to teach in *Surya Namaskar* (Sun Salutation). The *ball* directions really help to interrupt chronic yoga patterns that often result in an overly arched lumbar from habitually sending the *ball* back when "back bending."

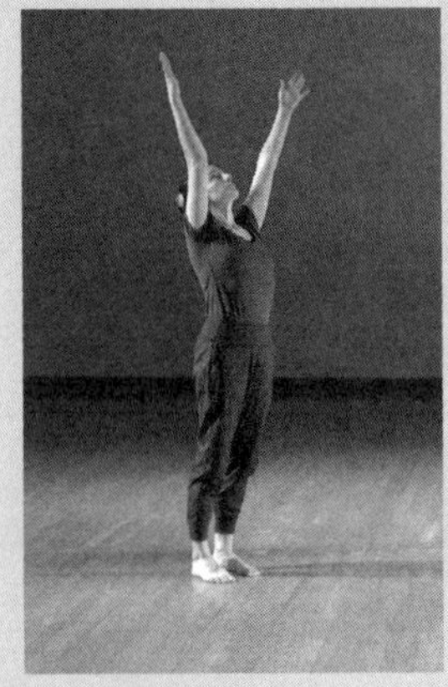

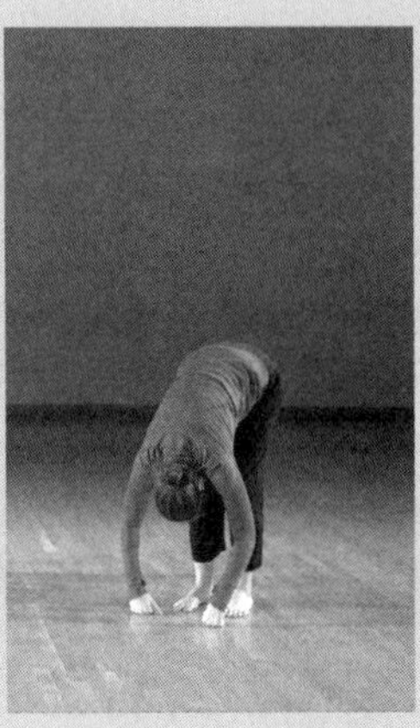

MOVEMENT EXPLORATION 17.1: ARMS REACHING ABOVE HEAD AND FOLDING OVER WITH BALL DIRECTIONS DISAFFINED AND AFFINED

Looking up, reach your arms overhead in *Urdva Hastasana* while directing the *ball* back with your weight toward your heels; how does this affect your breath, neck/jaw, hips, and ankles? Now try again but as you look up, allow the *ball* to go forward and your weight more toward your toes. How was that different in your breath, neck, jaw, and lower back in particular? Now do a similar experiment with a foward fold.

In this movement exploration, I hope that you noticed that sending the *ball* back actually exerted a downward force on the shoulders, upper chest, neck, and jaw, perhaps even causing the neck to feel strained (Primary patterning is disaffined with reaching up in space). Sending the *ball* forward facilitated the full Secondary pattern that is affined with reaching up into space. Affining Primary and Secondary throughout Sun Salutation can offer clear, whole-body directions and intents that make riding the flow of the sequence more organic, as well as free the breath.

If you are familiar with Sun Salutation A, taking time to consider the Simple Model throughout can be the first step in identifying habits that might be making the sequence less enjoyable to do. Each time there is a "majority" Primary pattern, is there any catching in Secondary that you can let go? An example might be that while you are in a forward fold, you keep shortening the cervical spine to see the mat instead of letting the crown of the head direct fully down to the mat, to instead see your shins (it is fully reasonable to bend your knees to allow the *ball* and hips to continue going back and up toward the ceiling, so the full Primary is accessible). When there is an overall Secondary intention, are you able to let go of Primary and surrender to the full opening of the front body as the *ball* directs forward? An example might be in cobra if there is a habit of resistance to opening the upper chest, clavicles, and throat. You might feel your cervical spine/neck overly active, trying to take on most of the arching (which might feel uncomfortable and diminish breathing), when the Secondary could be more shared throughout your whole spine.

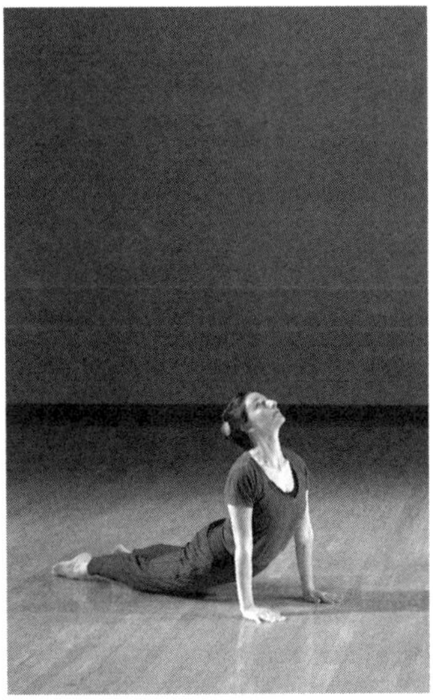

Video: Yoga

The Framework has also really influenced the way I approach plank pose (*Phalakasana*). This asana is ubiquitous in fitness, wellness, and dance contexts

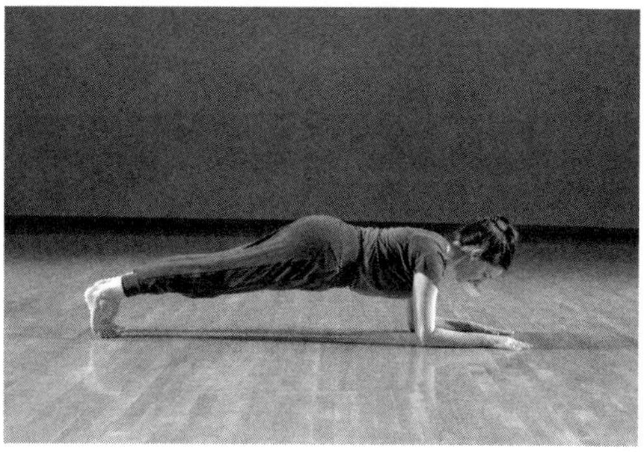

and is touted as a wonderful isometric whole-body strengthening exercise. The way I see it done by students in my dance classes, in yoga contexts, and beyond can be tough to witness. Responding to the body's orientation to gravity, all sorts of interfering habits emerge. Often, difficulty in achieving a solid plank position is attributed to a lack of upper-body strength. I submit that plank pose has less to do with strength and more to do with understanding the spiral musculature in efficient coordination. Plank often defaults to an overall Secondary patterning, with the face and thoracic and lumbar curves sinking below the shoulder blades, the pelvis's weight taking the whole body on a ride toward collapsing on the mat. Many practitioners engage fierce mental discipline to override discomfort, holding the pose by force of will, evidenced in locked elbows and excessive muscular tension. Thus, what should be a transitional pose—a way through to the next thing (say, flowing through *Chaturanga* to downward-facing dog)—becomes a dreaded, stalled moment requiring excess energy and extra movement initiation to get out of.

Video: Plank

Integrating the *ball* directions here is very helpful. The previously mentioned sagging Secondary habit would be inadvertently arching the spine and sending the *ball* forward (more *Seagulls* phase)—great for cobra or upward-facing dog but not so much for plank. Sending the *ball* and whole spine back toward the ceiling in a more overall Primary, as in the *Sandals* phase, hovers the whole front body back and away from the mat. Heading toward *Chaturanga*, the *ball* would *stay* up and back, lowering the face and upper chest to the mat first and the hips slightly after. One of my litmus tests for whether the whole body is orienting up and back in an overall Primary is to check whether the elbows can stay available and soft even while pushing away from the floor. An additional fun quiz is to see if, by continuing to send all the curves of the spine and the pelvis up and back with soft elbows, you can accomplish a little whole-body "hop," with the hands and toes simultaneously leaving and returning to the mat. Anyone who has ever seen a startled cat springing up off the floor with a rounded spine has seen this whole-body patterning taken into strong action. Some people tend to remain too Primary; in this case, looking up a little and then Resetting the head can usually lengthen the whole pose overall.

Though Sun Salutation is primarily in the vertical and sagittal planes, in most yoga classes, once that foundational sequence has been practiced in parts or its entirety, the asanas add what are called "twists," moving the body into a fuller three-dimensionality by adding the transverse plane. From the Framework's Complex Model, these asanas can be tricky if there is an emphasis on keeping the global joints "square" or symmetrical. I often hear encouragement to keep hips and shoulders equal in certain postures or to keep the lower base of the posture square while twisting the upper against it. An example of this would be in revolved chair pose (*Parivrtta Utkatasana*), where, as practitioners turn their torsos to bring one elbow of the prayer pose across their centerline to meet the opposite thigh or knee, they are encouraged to keep both hips square and the weight planted evenly on the feet.

In these rotated asanas, the Complex Model might fly in the face of some yoga orthodoxies, but when applied subtly, adding the concepts of weight shifting, the asymmetrical balancing of Primary and Secondary, and feeling how the loading of the spirals can unfurl with ease (Resetting) can transform a twist into a more authentic *spiral*, something the body is naturally meant and wants to do.

MOVEMENT EXPLORATION 17.2: REVOLVED CHAIR POSE WITH COMPLEX MODEL

On your mat, start in chair pose: feet together, knees and ankles deeply bent, with pelvis directing back in space (similar to a squat), torso long, and palms pressed together at sternum.

Move to revolved chair pose, maintaining the initial foundation but now looking right to move the left elbow across your centerline to the outside of your opposite thigh or knee. Always: keep breathing.

Things to think about:

- The left shoulder is coming around in Primary while the right shoulder is opening up in Secondary.
- Notice if the shoulders want to be "the same"—do they both want to stay in either Primary or Secondary?
- Even though you may have experienced instruction to avoid changing the hips, notice that your hips want to do the same as your shoulders, with the left hip coming around in Primary and the right hip opening up and back in Secondary. This direction can be applied very subtly.
- As you spiral to the right, shift your weight slightly to your left leg, so your left leg is bearing slightly more weight (Engaged) and your right leg slightly less weight (Resetting). Remember the Complex Model mantra: *Spirals transfer weight.*
- Sense the deep connections from opposite hips to shoulders, feeling in your body the large swaths of spiral musculature. You might notice the way your skin or shirt stretches long across your back from your right hip to your left shoulder while conversely wrinkling across your front from the same shoulder to hip. Try to let go of thinking of your upper body twisting against your lower body in two separate chunks.
- Coming out of the pose, let this deep spiraling undo itself by turning your head back toward the front of the room and shifting weight back down to your right foot. That loaded spiral *wants* to undo itself (Reset).
- Notice that your chair pose is in a new place—it changed (Reset) by going into and coming out of a spiral.
- Try it to the other side.

I feel so fortunate to have stumbled into the practice of yoga, and I offer deep gratitude to the many yogis, yoginis, teachers, and students who have contributed to this ocean of embodied knowledge over thousands of years in human history. I keep in mind the historical context: Yoga is "union"—an opportunity to engage through the body with what master Patanjali referred to as "mastery over the dynamic forces of the mind" (Tigunait). In my own evolving and ongoing practice, the Framework helps me to direct my thinking and work with entrenched habits of mind and body, including my harsh inner critic. Working through interferences and the noise of life to get to union is an ongoing practice, one that I hope to keep undertaking patiently, with great kindness toward myself and others. May the Framework information be a rich, continued source of embodied wisdom that helps you in your practice and on your path. Namaste.

Elizabeth Johnson is a performer, choreographer, educator, Laban Movement Analyst, Certified Teacher of the Alexander Technique, and Registered Yoga Teacher. She teaches and presents nationally and internationally on dance and somatic pedagogies that highlight developmental movement, prosocial/trauma-informed education, and critical perspectives. From 2004 to 2017, her company, Your Mother Dances, featured her choreography and produced other national artists. Johnson has coauthored/authored three book chapters featuring Alexander Technique and developmental movement applications. She is an associate professor and chair of the Department of Dance at the University of Maryland, Baltimore County.

Exploring Three-Dimensional Connections in Tai Chi Chuan through Framework for Integration

Phyllis Richmond

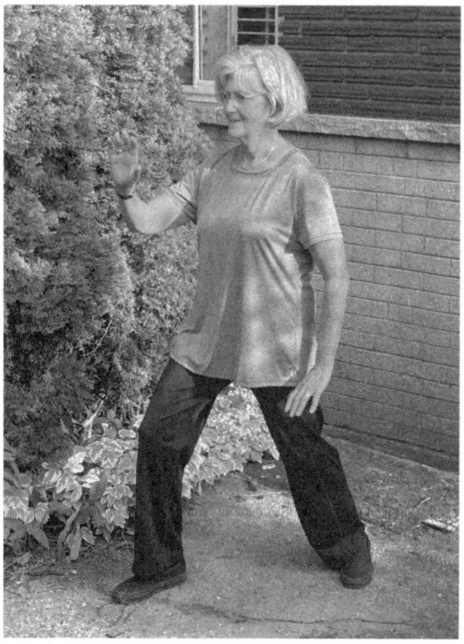

I came to Framework for Integration as an Alexander Technique teacher, a Certified Laban Movement Analyst, a former dancer, and a longtime student of Tai Chi Chuan. Over the years, the Framework has percolated into my understanding of both everyday movement and specific activities. Here are a few thoughts about how Framework for Integration has informed my exploration of the working of the body in Tai Chi Chuan training.

Although this way of analyzing and describing movement is, obviously, not part of Tai Chi Chuan, aspects of Framework for Integration, such as Primary/Secondary curves and spirals, helped me understand the changing arrangement of my limbs and torso—bones, muscles, and fascia—in a coherent pattern as I learned the form. I was especially fascinated by the interplay of spirals within the form, and I spent time playing with the continuous alternation of Engagement and Reset in the spirals.

For example, in the brush knee posture, which is performed a bit differently in different styles of Tai Chi, the body faces the left cardinal direction—if you use the clock face, this direction would be 9 o'clock. The right arm is extended in front of the right shoulder, and the left leg is forward and flexed at the knee. The left hand is by the left hip and the right leg is extended back in what could be called, in the dance world, a lunge. Within that pose, there's a diagonal connection running from the right hand to the right shoulder down and around the back to the left buttock and down the left leg to the foot on the floor—this can be seen as a Primary. The connection from the left hand and shoulder runs across the front of the body to the right hip and down the right leg to the right foot—a Secondary. These curves cross as they wind around the body. I experience them together, one spiral against another, shifting and supporting the body in movement.

Tai Chi is not static; we have to move into and out of brush knee. Moving into brush knee, we can start facing front—12 o'clock—with weight on the right foot and toes of the left foot close to the right foot. Both legs are outwardly rotated. The left hand is near the right hip, and the right hand is near the right shoulder, with the elbow down. A Primary spiral runs from the left hand up to the left shoulder, across the back to the right hip and down to right foot. And a Secondary spiral runs from the right hand and shoulder across the front and down to the left hip and foot. To start moving, the right leg (hip, knee, and ankle) bends, and the left foot extends to the left and back to reach toward 7 o'clock. We can allow pressure from the right foot on the ground to stimulate the Secondary spiral connecting through the body all the way to the left hand. The weight gradually transfers to the left foot, while the torso gradually rotates to face 9 o'clock, and the left hand is carried to the side of the left hip. Meanwhile, as the body turns and the weight transfers, the Primary spiral Resets, then Engages so that it runs from right hand to left foot. The Primary and Secondary exchange diagonals! We settle briefly into the brush knee posture, then move into the next Engagement/Reset to continue the sequence.

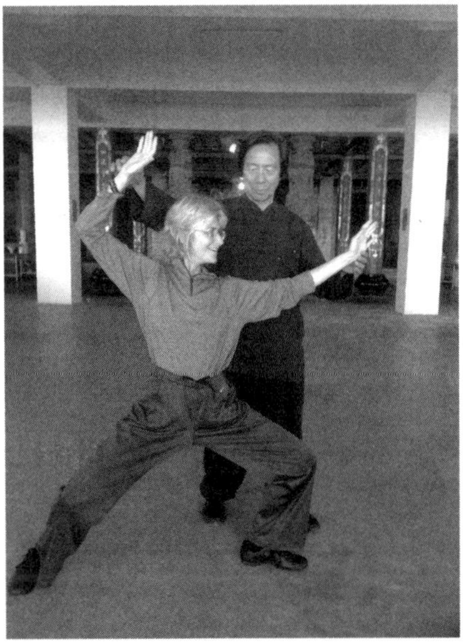
Phyllis Richmond with her teacher, Su Chin Piao

Each movement contains the seeds of the next; they are intertwined. When I was learning the form, Framework for Integration helped me clarify the body's changing three-dimensional organization during the sequence of linked movements. Three-dimensional thinking helped me experience the spiral stretches playing through the body, both creating and created by the ongoing movement. Now, as time has passed, I don't separate out the

Framework, but instead—in the context of all the other things I've learned about Tai Chi—experience more of the Integration!

Phyllis Richmond is a Certified Alexander Technique teacher, Certified Laban Movement Analyst, former dancer, and serious student of Tai Chi Chuan. She taught Alexander Technique for many years in North Texas: in the Theater Division of the Meadows School of the Arts, Southern Methodist University, Dallas, and in the College of Music at the University of North Texas, Denton. In addition, she has taught many workshops and master classes for universities and professional training programs in Texas, Oklahoma, Illinois, and abroad. Phyllis now lives and teaches in Evanston, Illinois.

Meditation Sitting: Movement That Clarifies Stillness

Luc Vanier

I began meditating in 1999 in my mid-thirties after starting to train as an Alexander Technique teacher. Within the process came the need to learn about and address certain mental habits. My psychotherapist at the time, Patrick, mentioned that I might benefit from gaining some awareness in my life. That observation proved truer than I ever could have imagined. A generous mentor, Sally, helped me first get acquainted with the practice of the Four Pillars of Mindfulness.

While there is no expectation that a practitioner must sit on a cushion, as a chair would serve *sitting* just fine, most of us do try. Sitting on a cushion close to the floor is akin to squatting. It is an extreme version of our usual sitting in a chair. For me, the activity was an ordeal, and while most people would expect a professional dancer to have the flexibility to facilitate *sitting* in meditation, this was not the case. I struggled, especially as I started to do retreats with multiple sessions a day.

As I was learning to teach the Alexander Technique through a developmental lens, it was also clear that for me, the traditional meditation posture would not happen all at once. The body–mind would need time to open after years of closing itself up. F. M. Alexander's principle of *psychophysical unity* as discussed in Chapter One maintains that the body and mind are inseparable. Traditional directions for sitting often seem to divide the practitioner into body parts; often there are directives for paying attention to positions of the legs, hips, spine, head, gaze, and hands, for example. Then, after giving such specific parameters, many teachers will turn around and emphasize that the body and mind are actually inseparable. This can be confusing, especially to beginning practitioners who have gone to great effort to "arrange" themselves "the right way" to begin meditating.

The problems can escalate if we confuse the physical directions that are given to us. I remember an experience from my early years when, in hearing that I should sit "still," I tried to do just that, only to find my skin flushed, heart rate elevated, and whole body numb from exertion after forty-five minutes. The experience taught me I was not going in the right direction. I was trying to split myself into body and mind, one over the other, a common problem in our current era. The answer was to connect my somatic awareness to my sitting.

Somatic practices (work that allows us to perceive our experience from an AQAL Individual/Subjective perspective—refer to Ken Wilber's work in Chapter One) have had some impact on sitting posture in recent years. A meditation leader may start sessions with advice such as "*do* this with your pelvis and then *do* this with your spine and then *do* this with your . . . etc." Unfortunately, these directions are often misinterpreted, since most of us are operating with, as Alexander said, *unreliable sensory appreciation,* where what we think we are doing may not be what we are actually doing. Our bodies continually readjust the *feeling* of the relationships of various parts—a map of our reality of self in which we feel this self as "normal." When we trust these feelings without question, we enter a vicious cycle of faulty sensory reality that only reinforces the relationships instead of freeing them up.

When faced with confident instructions about how to correct posture, we will likely attempt to *do* the directions instead of removing the obstacles that would allow for a freer, more upright posture. For example, one of the most misunderstood directions can be to *relax.* This promotes us trying to perform what we *feel* is relaxation, which from an outside eye might look like slumping. In some cases, consciously following the provided directions will have good results, but only temporarily, as habits easily take over the minute one stops maintaining clear intent in a new direction. Also, for us to assume that we could find one perfect position that would be good for all situations is misguided. As mentioned in Chapter Eleven: Breathing, one breath alone will change our whole body.

The somatic guidelines provided by the Framework center around our sense of movement (kinesthesia) and the fact that our brains were created to coordinate movement. It is not about looking to experience our body from skeletal, nervous, digestive, or circulatory systems, all of which are important. Rather, the Framework looks to first integrate our kinesthesia with various body systems so they become part of our daily experience of movement and consequently facilitate further introspection. The simplicity of the Framework's approach encourages deeper and deeper levels of somatic inquiry and support.

Seven Points Posture Translated Through the Framework

Keeping the above in mind, it is important to listen to the traditional directions, sometimes referred to as the *Seven Point Posture of Vairocana,* without directly enacting them. This is important: Do not react to perceived commands. What you are presently doing is most likely fine in and of itself. Oppose the urge to judge yourself. Second, as we contemplate these directions, we can analyze whether a Primary or Secondary is being suggested, and with an understanding of our habitual patterning, we can redirect the activity lightly, always toward simplicity.

Generally, from a Simple Model perspective, we know that *sitting* will require an overall Primary, especially in the hip joint. The direction asking that we sit with our "chin slightly lowered" calls for a release of the head forward on top of the spine, which is also a suggestion to allow for a Primary at the top of the spine. With the instruction that the shoulders should rest evenly, those with uneven spines might feel like they need to move the shoulders into place instead of addressing the asymmetrical habits inherent in spirals. At this point, addressing the lengthening of the spine is probably more useful than trying to *level, open,* or *relax* the shoulders.

In the command asking that the "body should not be bent forward or backward, but kept straight," the spine is encouraged to be long between the hip and head, calling for a general extension in Secondary. Sometimes the best way to know if you are "bent forward" is to actually bend forward with intent and then let it go. How did that feel? Do it again and now think of Engaging in Primary coming forward and Resetting toward Secondary coming out of it. Now do the opposite: Look up, and as the instructions say, "bend backwards." Do you have a preference? If doing this in sitting posture is too complex, try it lying down on the floor on your back. Look down at your chest, almost like a sit-up, and then let go; look up to the ceiling and slightly behind you and let that go.

To extend their spines, meditators who do not know of their habitual tendencies might overexert their lumbar spine (in Secondary) and/or pull their shoulders back, often not noticing that their upper back is not actually lengthening but rather staying in Primary (bending forward). If they tend to overly arch their spines in Secondary, they might unwittingly try to fix the issue by making their head/neck area overly Primary (chin tucked down and back). Being clear about our habits and how we plan to redirect them takes some somatic awareness.

Other directives, often coming from the practice of yoga, ask for the knees to touch the floor, creating a tripod with the pelvis while sitting slightly forward on the cushion. From a Complex Model perspective, the open, outwardly rotated legs are in Secondary while the seated pelvis is in Primary (dual counterspirals). Even though the position is extreme for most of us, it is in balance between Primary and Secondary. Without a Reset of your lower back's Secondary, your legs will not be encouraged to open in Secondary. A higher seat allowing for a more comfortable Primary of the lower back and adjusted cushions under the knees might help you continue to direct the knees' opening in Secondary without forcing the hip joint or lower back. Another approach might be to sit as if on a saddle on top of a cushion, with the hips releasing in Primary and the knees releasing forward and away from the hips in a slight Secondary rotation (as on a horse).

Four Phases on the Cushion

Let's notice where your *ball* might habitually want to go while sitting in meditation. Three types of habits can usually be observed in meditators: 1) continually sending the *ball* back, 2) continually sending it forward, or 3) the pelvis becoming passive as it receives the weight of the torso. Before we can address the *ball*, notice the actions of the hands and arms. In *sitting*, the hands are usually supported on the knees, on your lap, or in a mudra (gesture) such as a prayer position with the two hands together. Noticing whether the arms are at play and whether they are pulling (Secondary), pushing (Primary), or not participating (held) will help free up the legs and get the *ball* moving (refer to Movement Exploration 11.5: Upper and Lower Triangles in Breathing).

When first becoming acquainted with these movements on the ball, we advocate for a playful, rather exaggerated approach. But on the cushion, these movements can be performed in an imperceptible way, so that no one would even notice that you are moving. You can review Movement Exploration 7.3: Four Phases Adding Limb Directions and extrapolate the movements on the ball to a more subtle version while sitting, being mindful of simply allowing the movement to happen, rather than controlling it.

MOVEMENT EXPLORATION 17.3: FOUR PHASES ON THE CUSHION

Once you can feel your arms' habitual action, it's easier to reorient the *ball* in relationship to intent on the cushion by going through an adapted "micro" version of the Four Phases:

1. First, let your head release forward on the spine and allow the whole spine from the neck to the tail to soften (*Sandals*—Primary Ball Back). While doing this, allow the head to take you forward in space from the hip joint by a small bit. The arms are Resetting.
2. Then, slowly start to look up with your eyes, allowing the whole body to gently respond in support (*Ocean*—Secondary Ball Back). The arms are pulling into Engagement.
3. Then, give up most of the intent to look out, and while keeping this newly found length, simultaneously let yourself come back to upright with eyes looking up (*Seagulls*—Secondary Ball Forward). The arms are Resetting.
4. Then rest easy, letting the eyes Reset to the horizon (*Beach Chair*—Primary Ball Forward). The arms are Engaging in Primary, freeing your legs.

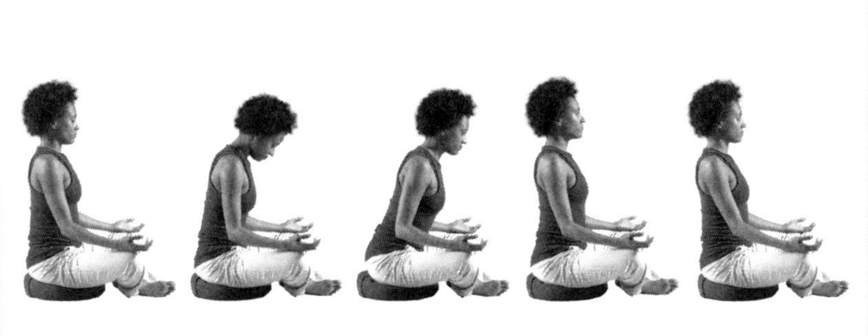

Video: Meditation Sitting

Recuperating

I find that a clear preparation will lead to a more informed, less reactive awareness of the body while sitting. If at any time you are getting tired in your sitting position, consider using the spirals to rest. For example, slowly look behind yourself with your eyes, sequentially allowing the neck to change and the weight to transfer, and then let the shoulders, hips, and knees follow. Having reached the end of the spiral, give up the intent to look around and let your hips lead you back to sitting naturally and effortlessly.

When fatigued, it is traditionally encouraged to stand and walk. Keep in mind that your habits will follow. Sometimes the best thing you can do is lie on your back with knees bent and a support behind your head (such as a thin book or rolled-up towel). As in *sitting*, the intent is not to hold on or create extra tension, but rather, to peel away the layers of habits to reveal the possibilities that have been there all along, reinvigorating our natural capacity.

> Please take what is useful and leave the rest behind. I am ever grateful to my teachers of Dharma and value highly their presence in the world. Any faults in interpreting the classic directions are mine alone.
>
> —Luc Vanier

Luc Vanier teaches somatic classes at the University of Utah. As a pedagogue and integral researcher, Luc has lectured and presented his research extensively nationally and internationally, and his cowritten book *Dance and the Alexander Technique* was published by the University of Illinois Press (in Spanish with Pequeña Hoja). He founded the Integral Movement Research Center and co-created Framework for Integration.

Chapter 18

Guest Contributions—Clinical/Therapeutic Applications

The authors of the three essays in this chapter have considered how the Framework concepts can be useful in therapeutic settings. These applications reflect the wide-ranging efficacy of the Framework in thinking about such things as fear-avoidance behaviors, joint hypermobility, chronic pain, and trauma recovery.

Thoughts on the Framework's Clinical Applications

Nikki Marini

I believe the primary way that the Framework can be useful in a therapeutic setting is by helping patients and clients explore and recognize their habitual movement patterns. The work facilitates self-awareness about areas of muscle tension, stiffness, hypomobility, or decreased range of motion. This awareness can help clients understand the rationale for their individual treatment plans and increase self-efficacy. When combined with specific treatments to address impairments, the Framework has the potential to improve patient outcomes.

The work can also be used as a safe way to help introduce movement to patients with fear avoidance behaviors, or for those beginning to introduce specific movement in one plane of motion after an injury. Also, it can be used as a gentle way to downregulate the sympathetic nervous system, self-mobilize, and improve carryover between sessions.

The ball work magnifies feedback to the patient about habitual and/or faulty movement patterns, as well as inefficient posture. The Framework's ball work could also be useful in the clinic before teaching stability work on the ball, as a way to emphasize the concepts of mobility and stability. Performing these bigger movements first, with awareness, could help highlight the areas we attempt to stabilize during more traditional ball work.

Overall, the Framework offers a safe way for clients to explore movement possibilities and gain understanding of their own unique habits and patterns.

Nikki Marini is a doctor of physical therapy with a clinical doctorate degree from the University of California San Francisco/San Francisco State University. Coupled with her physical therapy education, Nikki has a background as a professional dancer, yoga instructor, Pilates teacher, and licensed massage therapist. She also earned dual bachelor's degrees in biology and dance from the University of Illinois Urbana-Champaign (UIUC). Nikki was exposed to the Framework when she participated in Rebecca Nettl-Fiol's faculty course at UIUC.

Framework for Integration: Finding Connections in Hypermobility and Chronic Pain

Kym McDaniel

Joint hypermobility syndrome and chronic pain have defined my relationship with my body. Hypermobility definitions usually refer to someone who exhibits an extreme range of joint mobility and/or joint, tissue, or skin fragility. My relationship with physical hypermobility is easy to trace. My limbs were pulled out of their sockets often and early in my life, as well as pursuing dance, a medium that often gives attention and positive regard for high leg extensions and the ability to bend, twist, and contort into varying choreographies. Unsurprisingly, my career as a dancer was marked with chronic injuries.

When I was introduced to the concept of the mind–body connection, my curiosity about emotional hypermobility grew. If the mind and body are connected, is it possible that my mind is as flexible and expansive as my body? How does the hypermobile mind hold similar, limitless ranges as the hypermobile body, but this time manifesting in thought, emotion, and sensitivity? I remembered how, as a young girl, I often emotionally shape-shifted into different roles, usually with the intention to please whomever I was around. The capacity to hold the emotions of everyone in the room felt natural to me. As an adult with the knowledge of trauma, I now understand how this was also a method of survival and self-protection.

As I trained to become an Alexander Technique teacher, my shape-shifting habits began unraveling. I realized how uncomfortable I was with physical and emotional self-advocacy, care, and boundaries. Although I had dealt with widespread chronic injury and pain for most of my life, during the time I was training to be an AT teacher, I sustained an unexpected head injury while performing on stage. The injury was the first time I realized how my pain, and therefore, my life, depended on speaking up for my needs.

People with invisible illnesses and/or disabilities are very often disbelieved by others who judge our symptoms or illnesses as "not real." A nondisabled public demands to "see" the disability to believe it for themselves. The paradox for people with hypermobility is that the disability is either invisible (to others) in our everyday lives or hyper-visible (like being praised in a dance class for high extensions).

As I negotiate pain and illness, Framework for Integration has provided a language for making conscious choices while in pain. I offer my experiences below with the awareness that each body experiences pain differently. My hope is for continued conversations integrating the Framework as a guide for play and relief, especially for people who are chronically ill, have disabilities, and live with pain.

Application: Shower Chair

In my dreams, I have a massive walk-in shower outfitted with waterfall shower heads and a wall-to-wall granite bench to sit on while showering. In reality, I have a plastic shower chair wedged inside a steel tub. In any case, my chair helps my heart rate stay low and avoid a POTS (Postural Orthostatic Tachycardia Syndrome) attack. My chair and compact tub provide an opportunity to practice Primary and Secondary, Engagements, Resets, and spirals on the *ball* (shower chair). As I reach for a hair product behind me, I look with my eyes and head, transfer my weight, and extend in a Secondary Ball Forward (*Seagulls*) to reach for the product. Grabbing the product, I Reset and unwind my spiral. Washing hair is a combination of Engagement and Reset until I repeat the process—look, turn and shift weight, extend and release product, unwind spiral. Eventually, I stand and rinse my hair—an Engagement. My chair waits nearby to facilitate rest and Reset.

Application: Swimming

In my late teens, I used to voraciously swim laps several times a week to "supplement" my dance training (aka control my weight). I had killer headaches almost every night I left the pool. A decade later, I tentatively entered the pool again, this time to experience weightlessness and pain relief. Facing the sky with my limbs extended like a giant starfish, I feel the small Engagements/Resets as my body adjusts to floating. My back is in Secondary, keeping my torso afloat, while I notice my head habitually pulling to engage in Primary against the overall Secondary (I have the opposite habit floating face down—my head pulls in Secondary against the overall Primary, triggering the old headaches). Now, floating on my back, I decide to relax the top of my head back into the water, which brings my body into an overall Secondary Ball Back (*Ocean*). The Reset of my neck is a relief. Without gravity interfering, I become as light as the air around me—the most gracious Reset.

Sometimes, I swim the length of the pool. In the moment of activity, the strong pulls of my historical lap swimming make slowing down and becoming curious difficult. However, at the end of the lap, my body lets me know what she needs. I tuck my knees and head into an extreme Primary. Curling into a ball, I sink under the water and feel joy.

Application: Appropriate Tension

As a child, I often negotiated hypermobile muscle fatigue by alternating between extreme Secondaries and Primaries. I especially remember moving between large spinal extremes when practicing the piano.

Recently, in an effort to find a hobby and "do something fun for once," I found a piano teacher and set up a lesson. For the first time in decades, I played a song memorized from childhood. Afterward, the teacher asked if I enjoyed playing the song. Surprised at the question, I replied, "Yes!" She then noted that while I played, my fingers and wrists drooped on the keyboard. My sagging wrists produced slurred notes and a sluggishness to the traditionally lively song. As she played an example note, I watched her hand lightly rebound on the key. At once, I was struck with the ease, lightness, and Reset of her hand. Ironically, while I had emotionally found pleasure in playing the song, my body was telling a different story. Now, when I sit at the bench, the activity has become less about playing notes and more about the mindfulness of discovering the pleasure and rhythm of reclaiming the past.

Becoming curious about my physical and emotional extremes, juxtapositions, and pain continues to be a lifelong journey. I find comfort in knowing that finding connection is an ever-changing, ongoing process with no limits or fixed ends. I know this to be true as it is mirrored every day in my own embodied hypermobile experience.

Kym McDaniel is a filmmaker, choreographer, curator, and educator. Her films have screened nationally and internationally in film festivals and galleries, and at conferences and universities. She was introduced to Framework for Integration as part of her AmSAT Alexander Technique training. She holds an MFA in Cinematic Arts, a BFA in Performance and Choreography, and a BA in Psychology from the University of Wisconsin-Milwaukee. She received an Advanced Certificate in Disability Studies from the City University of New York. She is an assistant professor in the Department of Dance at the Ohio State University.

Trauma Recovery and Dance Movement Therapy: Framework for Integration Applications

Sara Yanney

I have been pursuing somatic studies for over twenty years to find a deeper understanding of the human body and movement, the complexity of its beautifully evolved design, and how this affects the health of the mind and body. From the moment I was introduced to Framework for Integration and took classes from Luc and Elizabeth, I could tell they had something new to offer me that I had not yet found through other somatic studies. The concepts take time and patience, much like the Alexander Technique, but once the fundamentals of the Framework made sense in my mind and body, it brought me a new understanding of my own movement, how I teach dance and the Alexander Technique, and how I can support clients as a clinical health counselor and Dance/Movement Therapist. As well as helping me be healthier in my body, it has been crucial in my own healing of complex PTSD.

I had been studying Framework for about three years, and one day in the training course, Luc kept encouraging me to let go of some extra Primary I was holding on to between two vertebrae in my lumbar spine and allow them to release into length in Secondary. The moment my body listened and let go of this deeply ingrained habit, I had an overwhelming rush of emotion that made me sob uncontrollably. At the time, I did not understand why I had a strong emotional release from just letting go of some Primary in one small spot. After years of exploring the Framework more, studying somatic psychology, and learning more about the nervous system, I now know that due to early childhood trauma, I was holding on to Primary in that one spot as an armoring of protection when I was not safe. Because the spinal cord moves through the spine, it makes sense that emotional holding, our nervous system, and sense of safety are closely related to our habits around how we organize Primary and Secondary in relationship to the whole self.

In her book *Sensing, Feeling, and Action: The Experiential Anatomy of Body-Mind Centering*, Bonnie Bainbridge Cohen noted how when the body is in extension (which would be toward Secondary), the sympathetic nervous system becomes activated, "which relates to fright, fight, flight, or freeze reactions. It increases the heart rate, rate of respiration, and in general will channel blood flow away from the viscera and into the skeletal muscles and brain" (Bainbridge Cohen 2012, 16). When the body is actively in flexion (which could be toward Primary), this activates the parasympathetic nervous system. This means the whole self believes you are safe, sending blood flow to the organs, "which relates to digestive function, repair and recuperation" (Bainbridge Cohen 2012, 16). This helps to explain why many people with high anxiety or stress often have somatic symptoms such as digestive distress, with not enough blood flow going to the organs. After I went through a new traumatic event in my early thirties, I began to get kidney stones at least once a year. When I started studying the Framework through AT training along with personal work on managing stress, I stopped having kidney stones and have not had one in over five years. Learning how to balance my use of Primary and Secondary with the Framework helped me learn how to better balance the use of my whole self and, therefore, also my nervous system.

One of the concepts that distinguishes the Framework is the idea of Engagement and Reset within patterns of flexion and extension. This allows the sequence of the Four Phases to be not just a series of shapes imitated in the body, but a way of organizing the body in movement. If one can follow this cycle of Engaging and Resetting, there is never a moment of collapse. I used to have habits of collapsing in both Secondary and Primary because of both my hypermobile body and my patterns of holding trauma in my spinal organization. Exploring these patterns with the whole self involved, without any collapse, helped me find more ease in my body and my mind. Applying the Framework concepts opened my body to finding its natural poise and organization, which then helped open my whole psychophysical self to healing early childhood trauma that I had not been able to unravel until I could understand the Framework more fully in my mind and body.

Using Framework for Integration in the Therapy Session

As a practicing Dance/Movement Therapist, I frequently see how the Four Phases are active in clients' use, and I use the Framework to help them with healing trauma and balancing their nervous system for holistic wellness. One of the benefits of working with children, even those who have experienced complex trauma, is that often, they are still more connected to their bodies and less shy about moving. In my office space, I provide props that encourage movement, specifically the Four Phases, so my patients have tools to help them experience and trust their bodies and movement instincts, depending on what they need in that session.

With the physioball, clients instinctually cycle through Primary and Secondary as they sit on the ball. They also like to roll over the ball or "surf" on the front surface of their bodies, forward and back in the sagittal plane, which also allows a cycling through the Four Phases but in another orientation.

Another prop I use is a "hopper" ball—a large ball with a handle to hold on to—and as my patients bounce, they instinctually and interestingly cycle through the Four Phases in what can be called *Accelerating Time* in the Laban/Bartenieff Movement Analysis system. The "crash pad" in my office (a kind of giant, flat, bean bag designed for kids who need sensory input and a place where they can land softly as they channel big energy into big movement) also allows clients to explore the Four Phases in various ways. The many possibilities of flipping, jumping, flying, and landing all require variations of cycling through Primary and Secondary and all directions on the *ball.*

Many clients with complex trauma will enter the room and immediately start doing these movements for at least the first five minutes of a session, just to allow some trauma and emotion to move through the body and sympathetic nervous system to get them to a more regulated place where they are ready to talk. Some clients I have may spend an entire session continually exploring variations of the Four Phases, especially early in the healing and therapeutic process.

Framework for Integration provides me an additional lens through which I can observe my clients' movement habits, preferences, and patterns, which tell at least some of the story of the traumas they have endured. Using the Framework, I gather information that helps me to see and support their immediate needs in session, as well as design longer-term plans that address and sustain their continued healing and agency.

Sara Yanney is a Dance/Movement Therapist and dance artist. As a therapist, she primarily works with children who need support with physical outbursts of emotion and healing complex trauma. As a performance artist, she is the director of the Equilibrium Dance Project based in Colorado. Sara received her MFA in Dance from the University of Wisconsin-Milwaukee, GL-CMA in Laban Movement Analysis from Columbia College-Chicago, and her MA in Somatic Psychology: Dance/Movement Therapy (MA, LPCC, R-DMT) from Naropa University, where her thesis was on applying Framework for Integration to help heal early childhood trauma.

Epilogue

It has been several years since Joan and Alex Murray moved from Urbana, Illinois, to London. Yet at ninety-four years of age, they continue to be curious, to get excited about making new discoveries . . . perfecting, maturing, refining their understanding of their lifelong work teaching the Alexander Technique. Joan continues to teach students all over the world via Zoom, limited to one student per day, and I am lucky enough to be able to Zoom with her occasionally. In a recent lesson with her, in her characteristic way with excitement and wonder, she wanted to show me what she had been working on. She had been watching a slow-motion video of a sparrow taking flight. And this stimulated her to create a movement exploration that teaches the principles that she saw in action in the bird.

—Rebecca Nettl-Fiol

Not perfection as a final goal, but the ever-enduring process of perfecting, maturing, refining is the aim of living.

—John Dewey, *Reconstruction in Philosophy*

MOVEMENT EXPLORATION E1: JOAN'S BIRD TAKING FLIGHT

From a seated position, make fists with both hands, and place them on your sternum. Then follow the sternocleidomastoid muscle, which goes from the sternum up to the back of the ears. If you turn the head to one side or the other, you can sense how much the head is involved, all the way from the top, to where your fingers are, down to your ankles. Now look down, and continue until you feel the weight of your head and shoulder girdle, and then continue curving forward as far as is comfortable. Now slide the fists down, following the sternocleidomastoid, to bring them underneath your armpits. Go on sliding your fists around your torso to meet behind the back. Look to your right and bring the right arm out to the side, keeping the fist, and continue turning until you can feel, or sense, your feet turning. Then take the other arm out to the side, looking at that fist as you do so, again, sensing your feet turning to adjust. Then finally, let the spiral to the left continue to take

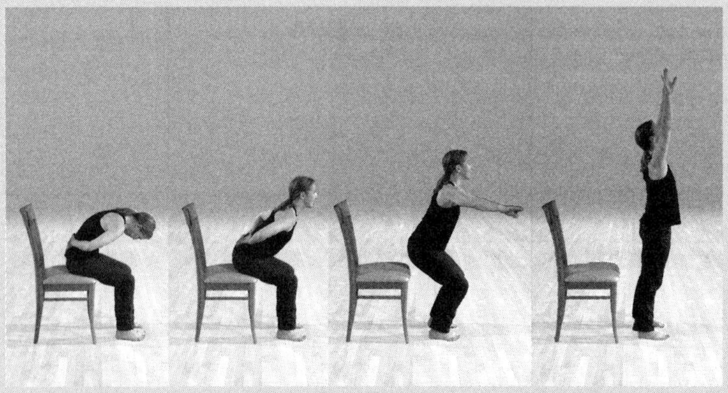

you up to sitting upright, with both arms coming overhead and pronated (backs of hands touching each other, releasing the fists). Bring the two arms down the front of the body, with the backs of the hands touching, until they separate, to bring the hands again under the armpits, fingers pointing downward as you slide the hands down your back. Incline forward until you're about to tip off the chair. Look up and stretch your fingers down as comfortably as you can. Finally, when you feel the time is right, swing yourself up with your arms until you come off the seat to stand up, with arms up as if you are taking off in flight.

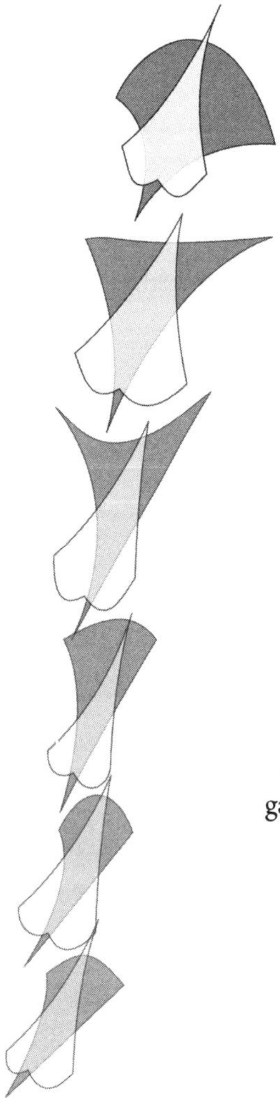

For us, this validated our work on the Framework, which began as a means of making an organizing system that would explain the brilliance of Joan's teaching and Alex's vast knowledge of the principles of Dart's work in relation to the Alexander Technique. Here was a clear demonstration of the Triangles in action, where the base of the Upper Triangle (shoulder girdle) provides support for the point of the Lower Triangle (neck), which emerges from underneath as the bird looks up.

> "When I was doing it, I could get more air it seemed. And I thought, what a clever little bird! It knew exactly when it could go—it was sprung. I just think it's so wonderful that a little bird can find it. It was looking—you could see the quivering—the energy of the stretch. It knew that it could gather air. With the spread of the fingers. It didn't work unless there was enough tone. It's extraordinary—that little bird got an arch all the way from here. And his little head, the more he looked up, the stronger you could see he could feel. And off he flew."
>
> —Joan Murray

We hope that you will engage in the never-ending process of perfecting, maturing, and refining. To find the spring, the energy of the stretch, the gathering of the air, the tone, and the strength to fly.

Supplemental Videos

Foreword

Interview with Luc and Joe

Chapter 2

Laban's Dimensional Scale

Chapter 4

Movement Explorations

4.6. Ballroom Walking Forward and Back with Your Hands Touching and Your Back in Primary
4.8. Primary Reset in a Chair
4.9. Primary Reset on a Bed

Extra Video

Shape Versus Movement—Using Straps to Look Up and Down

Chapter 5

Movement Explorations

5.4. Rolling from the Back to the Front
5.5. Spiraling to Standing
5.6. Counterspiral in a Chair
5.7. Walking
5.9. Double Spiral Straps
5.10. Mapping the Spirals of the Trunk
5.12. Fish Arms While Standing
5.13. Double Spirals of Arms—Upper Against Lower, Both Ways
5.14. Hip to Fingers Spiral Pathway
5.16. Spiral from Sitting with Legs in Front

Extra Videos

Mapping of the Trunk and Legs
Straps on Arms Double Spirals

Chapter 6

Movement Explorations

6.3. The Resilience of the Structure
6.5. Spiral Roll—Even and Organic Phrasing
6.6. Bouncing to Jumping
6.7. Walking in Twos and Threes
6.8. Sitting and Standing

Chapter 7

Movement Explorations

7.1. Getting Used to the Ball
7.3. Four Phases Adding Limb Direction
7.5. Circling

Extra Videos

The Four Linked Phases
Animated Four Phases

Chapter 8

Movement Explorations

8.1. Primary Control Illustration Lying Prone
8.2. Rocking Back and Forth on All Fours
8.4. Crawling on All Fours Revisited: Upper and Lower Triangles
8.5. Squatting with a Chair

Chapter 9

Movement Explorations

9.1. Primary Ball Forward (*Beach Chair*) with partner
9.1. Primary Ball Back (*Sandals*) with partner
9.2. Squatting Revisited with Triangle Animation
9.3. Baby in Squat Doing Lateral Shifts
9.3. Spirals in Transferring Weight While Standing

Extra Videos

Spiraling on the Floor with Illustrated Ball Direction
Triangle Engagement and Reset While Rollerblading

Chapter 14

Applications

Ladder Climbing
Getting in and out of a Car with Spirals
Walking with Primary and Secondary Spirals
Hammer
Riding the Bike
Skiing
Golf
Tennis
Kettlebell

Chapter 15

Application

A Basic Invert

Chapter 16

Application for Musicians:

When in Doubt, Up and Out

Coordination Underlying Musical Intention at the Harp, Part 1

Coordination Underlying Musical Intention at the Harp, Part 2

Coordination Underlying Musical Intention at the Harp, Part 3

Coordination Underlying Musical Intention at the Harp, Part 4

Coordination Underlying Musical Intention at the Harp, Part 5

Coordination Underlying Musical Intention at the Harp, Part 6

Coordination Underlying Musical Intention at the Harp, Part 7

Coordination Underlying Musical Intention at the Harp, Part 8

Coordination Underlying Musical Intention at the Harp, Part 9

Coordination Underlying Musical Intention at the Harp, Part 10

Coordination Underlying Musical Intention at the Harp, Part 11

Coordination Underlying Musical Intention at the Harp—
Synthesis plus Performance

Movement Exploration

16.1. Weight Transfer, Simple Spiral, Counter Spiral

16.2. Weight Transfer with the Violin

16.3. Circles

16.4. Figure Eight with the Violin

Extra Video

Using the Framework in Practice—A Video of the Process

Chapter 17

Applications

Yoga

Plank

Meditation Sitting

Glossary of Terms

Affinity—Borrowed from the LBMA system. Laban identified affinities, or correlations between the components of movement, which he defined as Effort, Space, and Shape. For example, he linked effort (qualitative) combinations with spatial directions for the most efficient performance. In the Framework, affinities can be thought of as factors that belong to or go naturally with a movement or intention.

Alexander Technique (AT)—A technique of mind-body reeducation, named after its developer, Frederick Matthias Alexander (1869–1955). The method teaches how to recognize and change undesired habits of movement and postural patterns, allowing for a more effective response to stimuli, and ultimately the achievement of better functioning.

Antagonistic Action—As used in F. M. Alexander's writings, the phrase refers to the stretch obtained when two parts are releasing away from each other. The term, as used in this book, implies a toning of the musculature, specifically the double-spiral musculature, eliciting coordination of the whole through a variety of oppositional forces.

AQAL: All Quadrants All Levels (Wilber)—A conception devised by philosopher Ken Wilber. The four quadrants refer to the most important dimensions of the Kosmos, namely, the interior and the exterior of the individual and the collective (Wilber 2000a, 42).

Ball Work—Activities performed on a physioball, designed to deepen awareness and coordination of the head-to-pelvis relationship.

Complex Model—The second layer in the Framework, this model recognizes our double-spiral musculature, reflecting the three-dimensional design of the human body.

Counterspirals—The interlocking of two spirals, where part of the body spirals in one direction, countered by another part spiraling in the opposite direction.

Dart Procedures—A series of developmental stages, outlined by paleoanthropologist Raymond Dart. This series of positions, when linked, becomes a movement sequence that retraces the path of development and evolutionary patterns.

Developmental Movement—The motor development of fetuses, infants, and babies as they learn to flex, extend, creep, crawl, sit, stand, and walk.

Direction (Alexander)—Deliberate, conscious thinking, guiding movement with intent. Directing your thoughts in such a way as to encourage the buoyancy and expansiveness that is inherent in the system.

Disaffinity—Factors that go against a movement or intention. (Opposite of affinity)

Double Spiral—Referring to the musculature of the human body, the double spiral is a complex interweaving of Primary and Secondary curves throughout the body in a double-helix design.

Effort (Laban)—One of the four main categories of analysis in the LBMA framework. Refers to the dynamic, energetic, and qualitative aspects of movement in four subcategories: 1. Weight: observed in the vertical dimension as the quality of decreasing pressure/lightness (up) and increasing pressure/strength (down); relates to sensing one's mass in relationship to the pull of gravity. 2. Space: observed in the horizontal dimension as how one attends to/focuses on their environment; toward crossing the body's midline is directing (which is specific/pinpointed), and away from the midline is indirecting (which is expansive and multi-focused). 3. Time: observed in the sagittal dimension as accelerating/quick (back) and decelerating/sustained (forward); are things speeding up or slowing down? 4. Flow: the underlying energetic nature of movement as seen in the qualities of freeing/unrestricted or binding/constrained.

Engagement—Muscular action.

Four Phases—Referring to four phases on the physioball. Includes Primary ball back, Secondary ball back, Secondary ball forward, and Primary ball forward.

Framework for Integration (Johnson, Nettl-Fiol, Vanier)—A co-created movement analysis system anchored in the ways babies and animals move that helps all movers make new, healthier movement decisions and encourages more coordinated and integrated bodily use.

Habit (Alexander)—Our unconscious responses or actions.

Inhibition (Alexander)—A refusal to consent to a habitually trained response. Taking a momentary pause to allow the space to bring a broader array of choices within our reach.

Integral Theory (Wilber)—A meta-theory or "philosophical map that brings together more than 100 ancient and contemporary theories in philosophy, psychology, contemplative traditions, and sociology" and "attempts to describe a framework for understanding and valuing the perspective of each theory and philosophical tradition and understanding how they relate to one another" (Duffy 2020). Wilber's purview "includes the essential perspectives of prerational, traditional, modernist, and postmodernist worldviews but also recognizes the limitations of each of these worldviews in addressing the increasingly complex challenges manifesting in the 21st century" (Duffy 2020). Includes AQAL and the Twenty Tenets.

Integrated Model—The third model in the Framework. This model looks at the relationship and responsiveness of the hips to the head and the head to the hips.

Intent—A thought, a wish, or a will to move toward or away from something.

Interference—What gets in the way of coordinated, easeful movement. Interferences most commonly occur through habitual movement or holding patterns of which we may be unaware.

Laban/Bartenieff Movement Analysis (LBMA)—A somatic system made of concepts from Rudolph Laban and Irmgard Bartenieff. Presents ideas of opposites to lay out a spectrum of qualitative possibilities for observing, describing, and analyzing movement. In this layered lens system, movement can be analyzed from distinct yet related categories (such as Body, Effort, Shape, and Space) as well as large polar ideas (such as Symmetry/Asymmetry, Inner/Outer, Function/Expression, etc.).

Layered Lens Model—A model that encompasses different lenses for looking at movement, each building on the previous one with more complexity. There is no contradiction between these models, but a deeper level of understanding emerges as one learns each subsequent model. Once understood, one may choose to view movement from any of the models.

Neutral—A place of non-moving equilibrium; a static model that connotes a correct way to stand, sit, or lie down, or to hold a particular body part, such as the pelvis or the spine.

Primary—The Primary curve is the curvature of the spine that is present in the fetus. The spine is in flexion; the hips, knees, and ankles are folded; and the arms are folded. Extending this into movement, any action toward flexion of the spine can be seen as going toward the Primary curve and would be called a Primary activity. (The opposite of Secondary)

Primary Control (Alexander)—The way in which our head/neck/back relationship leads and dynamically organizes the coordination of our whole body and all our movements.

Reset—Letting go of a muscular action. Finding something new as one lets go of an engagement, not to be confused with an opposite engagement.

Secondary—The opposite of Primary, the Secondary curves come about in development when the baby begins to look up. The spine goes into extension; the hips, knees, and ankles extend; and the arms pull. Any action toward extension of the spine can be seen as going toward the Secondary curve and would be called a Secondary activity.

Simple Model—From the Framework. This model looks at the two basic actions of the body: Primary, which moves toward the curve we were born in, and its opposite, Secondary, which takes us out of self and into the world.

Spiral—Refers to rotational movement of the body. Due to the double-spiral musculature of the body, a spiral movement sequences from the initiation point through the whole body, stimulating a weight shift.

Triangles: Upper and Lower—From the Framework, part of the Integrated Model. The triangles represent oppositional connections of the upper and lower body. The Upper Triangle's wide base is across the back and shoulder girdle, with the point at the sacrum/coccyx. The Lower Triangle's base is across the bottom of the pelvis, with the point at the occipital ridge. The overlaps in the triangles create strength built by opposition.

Twenty Tenets for Developmental Growth (Wilber)—Wilber's list of what he sees as trends and patterns common to evolutionary systems.

Unreliable Sensory Appreciation (Alexander) (or Faulty Sensory Appreciation)—The fact that one's kinesthetic sense can become unreliable due to habitual patterns of movement that "feel right."

Use and Functioning (Alexander)—The way you use yourself as you go about your activities affects your functioning, and, in turn, your functioning affects your use.

Whole Self (Psychophysical Unity) (Alexander)—The unity of body and mind. We are an indivisible whole. Every thought has a physical manifestation, and every action has a mental connection.

Bibliography

Aces Too High. n.d. "What ACEs/PCEs Do You Have?" https://acestoohigh.com/got-your-ace-score/. Accessed May 29, 2024.

Adrian, Barbara. 2008. *Actor Training the Laban Way: An Integrated Approach to Voice, Speech, and Movement.* Allworth Press.

Alexander, F. Matthias. 1984. *The Use of the Self.* Centerline (reprint of 1939 edition).

Alexander, F. Matthias. 1990. *The Alexander Technique: The Essential Writings of F. Matthias Alexander.* Edited by Edward Maisel. Thames and Hudson.

Alexander, F. Matthias. 1996. *Man's Supreme Inheritance.* Mouritz (reprint of 1946 edition, with additional material).

Alexander, F. Matthias. 2000. *The Universal Constant in Living.* Mouritz (reprint of 1946 edition, with additional material).

Alexander, F. Matthias. 2004. *Conscious Constructive Control of the Individual.* Mouritz (reprint of 1946 edition, with additional material).

Bainbridge Cohen, Bonnie. 2012. *Sensing, Feeling and Action: The Experiential Anatomy of Body-Mind Centering.* Contact Editions.

Bainbridge Cohen, Bonnie. 2018. *Basic Neurocellular Patterns: Exploring Developmental Movement.* Burchfield Rose.

Bartenieff, Irmgard, with Dori Lewis. 1982. *Body Movement: Coping with the Environment.* Gordon and Breach.

Batson, Glenna. 2009. "Somatic Studies and Dance." International Association for Dance Medicine and Science, resource paper.

Berman, Erica. 2017. *Sitting: The Physical Art of Meditation.* Self published.

Bernstein, Nicholai A. 1996. *Dexterity and Its Development.* Lawrence Erlbaum Associates, Publishers.

Bowman, Kevin J. 2009. "Holarchical Development: Discovering and Applying Missing Drives from Ken Wilber's Twenty Tenets." *International Journal of Transpersonal Studies* 28(1): 1–24. http://dx.doi.org/10.24972/ijts.2009.28.1.1.

Bradley, Karen. 2019. *Rudolf Laban.* Routledge.

Carrington, Walter. 1999. *Thinking Aloud: Talks on the Alexander Technique.* Mornum Time.

Dart, Raymond A. 1996. *Skill and Poise.* STAT.

De Alcantara, Pedro. 2011. *Integrated Practice: Coordination, Rhythm and Sound.* Oxford University Press.

Dewey, John. 1920. *Reconstruction in Philosophy*. Henry Holt and Company. Sourced from Project Gutenberg, 2012 ebook: https://www.gutenberg.org/files/40089/40089-h/40089-h.htm. Accessed May 29, 2024.

Duffy, James D. 2020. "A Primer on Integral Theory and Its Application to Mental Health Care." *Global Advances in Health and Medicine* 9. https://doi.org/10.1177/2164956120952733.

Eddy, Martha. 2002. "Somatic Practices and Dance: Global Influences." *Dance Research Journal* 34(2): 46–62. https://dynamicembodiment.org/library/articles/global influences.pdf. Accessed January 19, 2024.

Eddy, Martha. 2015. "The Ongoing Development of 'Past Beginnings': A Further Discussion of Relationships Between the Bartenieff Fundamentals of Body Movement and Perceptual-Motor Development Theories (Body-Mind Centering® and Kestenberg Movement Profile)." *SOMATICS: Magazine-Journal of the Bodily Arts and Sciences* 17(3): 18–32.

Eddy, Martha. 2017. *Mindful Movement: The Evolution of the Somatic Arts and Conscious Action*. Intellect.

Eddy, Martha, and Andrea Shakti Smith. 2021. *Dynamic Embodiment® and the Sun Salutation: Pathways to Balancing the Chakras and the Neuroendocrine System*. Handspring Publishing.

Glasford, Irene. 1970. *Rhythm, Reason, and Response, for the Musician, Pianist, and Teacher*. Exposition Press.

Goldberg, Marian, ed. 1996. *Beginning from the Beginning: The Growth of Understanding and Skill.* The Alexander Technique Center of Washington, D.C.

Graves, Clare W. 2005. *The Never Ending Quest.* ECLET Publishing.

Hackney, Peggy. 2002. *Making Connections: Total Body Integration Through Bartenieff Fundamentals.* Gordon and Breach.

Hanh, Thich Nhat. 1999. *The Miracle of Mindfulness: An Introduction to the Practice of Meditation.* Beacon Press.

Harvard University: Center on the Developing Child. n.d. "ACEs and Toxic Stress: Frequently Asked Questions." https://developingchild.harvard.edu/resources/aces-and-toxic-stress-frequently-asked-questions/. Accessed August 18, 2023.

Hutchinson Guest, Ann. 2005. *Labanotation: The System of Analyzing and Recording Movement*, fourth edition. Routledge.

Johnson, Molly. *Directing To Establish How Elements Relate to Each Other.* Lecture. AmSAT Virtual Annual Conference, June 25, 2022.

Johnson, Will. 1996. *The Posture of Meditation, First Edition.* Shambhala Publications.

Lahey, Jessica. "To Help Students Learn, Engage the Emotions." *New York Times*, May 4, 2016. https://archive.nytimes.com/well.blogs.nytimes.com/2016/05/04/to-help-students-learn-engage-the-emotions/.

Lama Pema Dragpa. 2018. "Seven-Point Posture of Buddha Vairochana." Padmasambhava Buddhist Center. https://www.padmasambhava.org/.

LaMothe, Kimerer L. 2015. "Recent Science Supporting 'Why We Dance': What Evidence Is There That 'I Am the Movement That Is Making Me?'" *Psychology Today*. https://www.psychologytoday.com/us/blog/what-body-knows/201510/recent-science-supporting-why-we-dance.

LaMothe, Kimerer L. 2015. *Why We Dance: A Philosophy of Bodily Becoming.* Columbia University Press.

Levine, Peter A. 2010. *In an Unspoken Voice: How the Body Releases Trauma and Restores Goodness.* North Atlantic Books.

Levine, Peter A., and Ann Frederick. 1997. *Waking the Tiger: Healing Trauma*. North Atlantic Books.
Menakem, Resmaa. 2017. *My Grandmother's Hands: Racialized Trauma and the Pathway to Mending Our Hearts and Bodies*. Central Recovery Press.
Mizrahi, Joseph. 2020. "Neuro-Mechanical Aspects of Playing-Related Mobility Disorders in Orchestra Violinists and Upper Strings Players: A Review." *European Journal of Translational Myology* 30(3). https://doi.org/10.4081/ejtm.2020.9095.
Mlodinow, Leonard. 2012. *Subliminal: How Your Unconscious Mind Rules Your Behavior*. Vintage Books.
Moore, Carol Lynne, and Kaoru Yamamoto. 1988. *Beyond Words: Movement Observation and Analysis*. Gordon and Breach Science Publishers.
Myers, Thomas. 2001. *Anatomy Trains*. Harcourt.
Myers, Thomas W. 2014. *Anatomy Trains: Myofascial Meridians for Manual & Movement Therapists*, 3rd ed. Elsevier.
Nettl-Fiol, Rebecca, and Luc Vanier. 2011. *Dance and the Alexander Technique: Exploring the Missing Link*. University of Illinois Press.
NPR, All Things Considered. June 17, 2014. "Your Brain's Got Rhythm, and Syncs When You Think." https://www.npr.org/sections/health-shots/2014/06/17/322915700/your-brains-got-rhythm-and-syncs-when-you-think.
Pacini, Adele M., and Philip J. Barnard. 2021. "Exocentric Coding of the Mapping Between Valence and Regions of Space: Implications for Embodied Cognition." *Acta Psychologica* 214. https://doi.org/10.1016/j.actpsy.2021.103264.
Preston, Valerie. 1963. *A Handbook for Modern Educational Dance*. MacDonal and Evans, Ltd.
Profeta, Vitor L. S., and Michael T. Turvey. 2018. "Bernstein's Levels of Movement Construction: A Contemporary Perspective." *Human Movement Science* 57: 111–133. https://doi.org/10.1016/j.humov.2017.11.013. Version of record for open access: https://www.sciencedirect.com/science/article/pii/S0167945717305717. Accessed May 21, 2024.
Roberts, Mady Shaw. October 6, 2017. "Why Do Conductors Always Conduct Ahead of the Beat?" Classic FM. https://www.classicfm.com/discover-music/why-conductors-beat-ahead/.
Rolland, Paul. 2007. *The Teaching of Action in String Playing: Developmental and Remedial Techniques*. Illinois String Research Associates (first published 1974).
Sacks, Oliver. 2008. *Musicophilia: Tales of Music and the Brain*. Vintage Books.
Schmidt, Richard A., and Timothy D. Lee. 2014. *Motor Learning and Performance*, 5th ed. Human Kinetics.
Shaw, Steven. 2007. *The Art of Swimming: A New Direction Using the Alexander Technique*. Collins & Brown.
Shubin, Neil. 2008. *Your Inner Fish*. Vintage Books.
Silver, Kagen S., and Amber K. Worthington. 2021. "Transtheoretical Model." In *Persuasion Theory in Action: An Open Educational Resource*. University of Alaska, Anchorage. Creative Commons Attribution-Share Alike 4.0 United States License. https://ua.pressbooks.pub/persuasiontheoryinaction/chapter/transtheoretical-model/.
Sweigard, Lulu. 1974. *Human Movement Potential: Its Ideokinetic Facilitation*. Dodd, Mead.
Thaut, Michael H. 2005. *Rhythm, Music, and the Brain: Scientific Foundations and Clinical Applications*. Routledge.

Tigunait, Pandit Rajmani. n.d. "Yoga Means Union, but Union with What?" https://yoga international.com/article/view/yoga-means-union-but-union-with-what/. Accessed July 29, 2023.

Vieuxtemps, Henri. 2002. *32 Etudes Opus 48*. Editio Musica Budapest.

Wahl, Colleen. 2019. *Laban/Bartenieff Movement Studies: Contemporary Applications*. Human Kinetics.

Wilber, Ken. 2000a. *A Theory of Everything: An Integral Vision for Business, Politics, Science, and Spirituality*. Shambhala Publications, Inc.

Wilber, Ken. 2000b. *Sex, Ecology, Spirituality: The Spirit of Evolution*, 2nd ed. Shambhala Publications, Inc.

Wilber, Ken. 2008. *Integral Life Practice: A 21st-Century Blueprint for Physical Health, Emotional Balance, Mental Clarity, and Spiritual Awakening*. Integral Books.

Winearls, Jane. 1968. *Modern Dance: The Jooss-Leeder Method*, 2nd ed. Billing and Sons Limited.

Index

LUC VANIER is the founding director of the University of Utah School of Dance and coauthor of *Dance and the Alexander Technique: Exploring the Missing Link.*

REBECCA NETTL-FIOL is a professor of dance at the University of Illinois at Urbana-Champaign and coauthor of *Dance and the Alexander Technique: Exploring the Missing Link.*

ELIZABETH JOHNSON is an associate professor and chair of the Department of Dance at the University of Maryland, Baltimore County.

The University of Illinois Press
is a founding member of the
Association of University Presses.

Composed in 10.5/14 Arno Pro Regular
with Avenir LT Std display
Text designed and composed by Kirsten Dennison
at the University of Illinois Press
Manufactured by Sheridan Books, Inc.

University of Illinois Press
1325 South Oak Street
Champaign, IL 61820-6903
www.press.uillinois.edu